Born FROM THE Heart

MY SURROGACY JOURNEY IN MEXICO CITY

Barbara van der Maaten

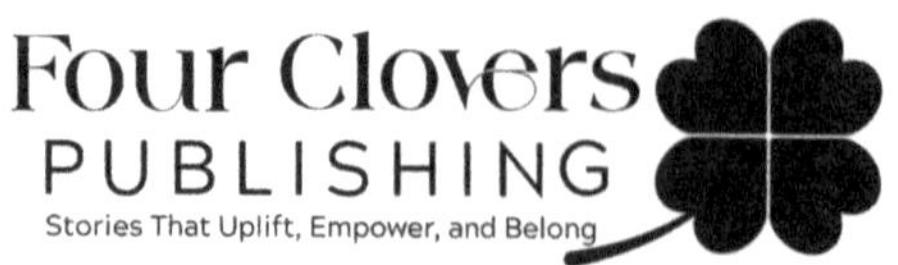

A Four Clovers Publishing Publication
Four Clovers Publishing Registered Offices: Caldwell, NJ 07006

Library of Congress Control Number: 2026905171

Barbara van der Maaten
Born From The Heart

ISBN: 979-8-9988858-4-6 (Print)
ISBN: 979-8-9988858-5-3 (E-Pub)
Published in the United States of America

Book cover and inside design by Kristin Broek
Editing and creative design consultation by Taryn Lagonigro
Professional photography by Fernanda Dames Photography & Kasia Strek Photography

Dedication

For Amalia, our miracle, and profound joy

You were loved and wanted long before you were born, and every step of this incredible journey was for you.

To Koen

Your steadfast love made the impossible possible. With my deepest gratitude, thank you.

Contents

Part I: Barbara's Journey

PART I
Barbara's Journey

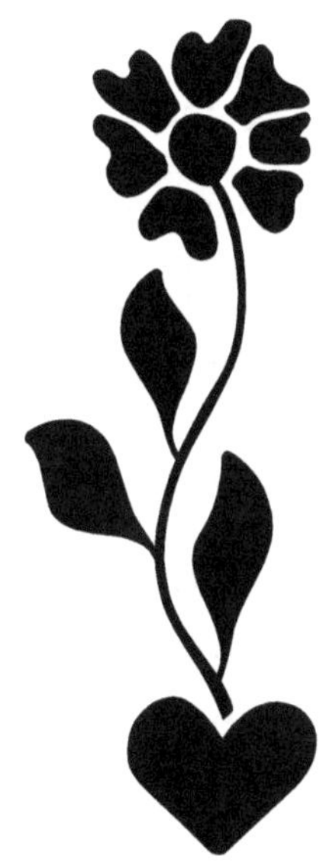

CHAPTER 1
The Dream Begins

I did not always know I would become a mother like this, but I always knew I would become a mother.

Whether it was through adoption or giving birth, that urge lived deep inside me. It was not a passing wish, but rather something I felt in my bones, a magnetic pull toward creating a lifelong bond with a child.

That desire only grew stronger as I became a Kindergarten teacher. Every day, I poured love and care into other people's children, helping them learn to read, resolving center time dramas, and watching tiny personalities bloom. I knew how to soothe a frightened child, how to spark their wonder, and how to be their safe place; but at the end of the day, I handed them back to their family and I went home with an ache, a dream, a yearning.

Watching other families form and grow all around me only made the ache stronger. It was not jealousy, but more of a longing. I wanted my own little hand to hold. I wanted to be the one tucking someone in at night, someone to call me "mama".

For years, I imagined this moment would happen for me. I was open to love; to building a family with someone else. But as time passed, life did not unfold in the tidy, linear way I had once expected. The traditional route of marriage, pregnancy, and then a baby, remained out of reach.

Still, the dream did not fade. If anything, it sharpened. I

began to ask myself harder questions: What if my life didn't have to follow the usual blueprint? What if motherhood could still be mine, just in a different shape?

Slowly, quietly, a new possibility began to take root. A possibility that would carry me across borders, across languages, across fears I did not even know I had. A possibility that would bring me to a foreign land, a possibility that would give me my child. I did not always know I would become a mother this way, but I always knew I would become a mother.

I met and married the love of my life, my husband Koen, at the ripe old age of thirty. We were full of adventure, joy, and curiosity about the world, so we traveled together for a few years, savoring our time as a couple. When we were finally ready to start our family, we did so with hopeful hearts.

There was no history of infertility in my family or in my husband's. We assumed, like so many do, that it would happen easily. That we would make a plan, take the right steps, and life would simply follow along, but that's not what happened.

Month after month, the silence of not conceiving grew louder. At first, we shrugged it off. Stress, timing, travel were our explanations. But as the calendar pages turned, our optimism began to slip into anxiety. Tests followed. Then more tests, and slowly, painfully, the truth emerged: the path to parenthood would not be simple.

The heartbreak of that realization was a quiet kind. It did not look like a tragedy from the outside. But it chipped away at the inside, at dreams, at confidence, at the belief that things would fall into place.

Still, I held on to the dream. Even as the path grew unfamiliar and uncertain, I never let go of the core truth I carried in me: I was meant to be a mother and maybe, just maybe, there was another way. We decided to seek help and made an appointment with a fertility specialist in our city.

What followed was a blur of ultrasounds, blood tests,

exams, waiting rooms, and clinical jargon. I was poked and prodded, inside and out, but the physical invasiveness was not the hardest part, it was the emotional coldness. Our fertility doctor had zero empathy. She delivered the news like she was reading the weather: detached, indifferent.

"You have diminished ovarian reserve," she said flatly. "You also have endometriosis and invasive fibroids." I sat there, stunned, as the words landed like sharp daggers. She continued: "Your only real option is to use donor eggs. And given your situation, you'll also need a surrogate." Diminished ovarian reserve meant that I had hardly any eggs left and was basically going into early menopause. Endometriosis is a condition where the lining of the uterus grows outside of the uterus and this can grow anywhere in the body. Invasive fibroids are basically uterine tumors that are not cancerous and tend to grow in size with time.

Just like that, the path I thought I was on evaporated. I did not cry then, not in that room. I felt too numb. Later, I cried in the car. I cried at home. I cried for the loss of the biological connection I had imagined. I cried for the mother I thought I would be. What I had to grieve was not just a diagnosis, it was the loss of a dream I had quietly carried all my life. I had to say goodbye to the idea of seeing my own eyes in my child's face. I had to mourn the chance to feel he or she grow inside me; to carry her through morning sickness and kicks and cravings.

There is a particular kind of ache that comes with letting go of your genetics and your body's role in the story. It is invisible to the world, but it cuts deep. That grief was real and I gave myself permission to feel it fully. I went to therapy to help me process that loss, because it was a loss - a very real one - and it deserved to be acknowledged, not brushed aside. Therapy gave me a place to speak the unspeakable parts, to release the guilt, and to eventually make peace with a new vision of motherhood.

However, beneath the grief, something else stirred; a tiny

flicker of hope. If this was the only way forward, then so be it. I was not giving up. I was not letting go of the dream. I would not carry my baby in my womb nor would he or she have my genetics, but I would carry and love my baby in every other way that mattered.

CHAPTER 2
Choosing Surrogacy

There is a strange stillness that follows devastating news. After that fertility appointment at our clinic, the world seemed quieter. We walked through our days in a kind of fog; measured, gentle, unsure. There was no roadmap for what we were feeling. I kept replaying her words: "You'll need donor eggs… and a surrogate." Two sentences that changed everything. However in truth, surrogacy was not our next step. Before that door even opened, we tried another path: adoption.

At the time, surrogacy felt entirely out of reach, especially financially. It simply was not an option. So we turned to what felt more feasible, and what had always been close to my heart: adopting a child who needed a home. We signed up with a licensed adoption agency in Canada, hopeful and ready to become parents in any way we could. We first pursued international adoption, starting with Ethiopia. We gathered documents, began the long list of required steps, and started to dream again. However, just as we were preparing our paperwork, Ethiopia shut down international adoptions. We were disappointed but not defeated. We pivoted next to Haiti—only to be met with more heartbreak. Rising civil unrest and political instability forced the process into indefinite suspension. So, once again, we pivoted, this time to domestic adoption in Canada. We went through the entire process twice: home studies, training sessions, reference checks, paperwork. We did it all and then we waited.

Four and a half long years passed. After all that time, after years of hoping, praying, and checking our phones with every email alert, one cold January morning we received a quiet, crushing update from the agency: We were still number forty-two on the waitlist. I remember sitting with that number like it was a rock on my chest. Forty-two. After everything we had done. That moment was both devastating and clarifying. We realized we could not keep waiting passively for our lives to begin. The door was not fully closed, but it was barely cracked open and we needed another way forward.

Slowly, we started looking into surrogacy options. At first, we searched locally in Canada, assuming we would find an agency or clinic that could guide us through the process. We were quickly met with roadblocks: extremely long waitlists with an average of three to four years to match with a surrogate. We also looked into surrogacy in the United States, but their price tag was exorbitant. It felt like trying to enter a locked building without a key. That is when Mexico entered the picture.

I do not remember exactly how it started, maybe a news article from someone who had done it themselves, but I began to see stories of people who had gone abroad to build their families. Mexico City, in particular, seemed to come up again and again. We kept digging until we came across an agency called Gestacy, based in Madrid but with an office in Mexico City. Their website stood out immediately, not just for the services they offered, but for the tone: warm, clear, human. They seemed to understand that this wasn't just a clinical decision, but the most emotional choice of our lives.

I reached out, hesitantly at first, and the response came quickly, and with it, a wave of relief. For the first time since our diagnosis, I felt seen. The team at Gestacy was responsive, informative, and, most importantly, kind. They did not treat me like a number or a medical case. They treated me like a woman trying to become a mother. Still, the decision to pursue an international journey came with hesitation. We were scared - truly scared.

You hear horror stories in the news - stories of scams, abandoned babies, legal loopholes, intended parents stranded in foreign countries. There is a reason many people feel nervous about crossing borders to build a family; it is unfamiliar, complex, and at times, portrayed as risky.

We carried those fears with us. We talked about them, researched them, worried about them in the middle of the night; but the more we learned, and the more real people we spoke to, the more that fear began to soften. We did not feel like we were walking into a trap. We felt like we were walking toward a possibility, a hope. Gestacy answered every question, explained the legal framework in Mexico, and helped us understand each step of the journey before we committed to anything. That transparency began to build our trust in this path.

Around the same time, we also began looking into egg donation in Canada. That is when we connected with Her Helping Habit, a compassionate and highly respected egg donor program based in Vancouver. One of the things that stood out to us immediately was that they were a known donor agency, which was exactly what we wanted. We did not want this part of the journey to be anonymous or sealed off. We wanted openness, honesty, and the option for our future child to know where they came from, if and when the time felt right.

Her Helping Habit's approach was thoughtful and ethical, and I appreciated how they supported both intended parents and donors equally. For the first time, the idea of using donor eggs did not feel like a loss. It felt like a gift, an act of generosity that could help bring our child into the world.

With Gestacy guiding us on the surrogacy side in Mexico City and Her Helping Habit supporting us with egg donation in Canada, we began to feel something we had not felt in a long time: momentum.

Koen and I had some long, late night talks. This was not a decision we made lightly. It was layered with emotion, logistics, finances, and of course, risk, but at the core of it all, we kept coming back to one question: what matters more, how we get there, or that we get there at all? For us, the answer was clear. It was time to cross borders, time to open our hearts to another kind of journey and time to find the people somewhere out there who could help us bring our baby home.

CHAPTER 3
Building the Team

The first time we met our team in Mexico City, it felt like stepping into a new chapter of our lives; not just because we were beginning the process, but because for the first time in years, we felt hope backed by action. After so many false starts with infertility, adoption setbacks, and waitlists, it was surreal to finally be moving forward.

We had already been working with Gestacy from a distance, but now it was time to meet some of the people in person. We booked flights to Mexico City and arrived nervous, excited, and full of questions. The city itself was vibrant and alive, so different from the snowy, quiet streets of Calgary. The contrast was striking: this ancient city bursting with color and noise was where our future would begin.

Our first meetings were with the medical staff at Fertilidad Integral, the clinic in Mexico City where our embryos would be created and the staff at Gestacy . Everyone we met through Gestacy was calm, professional, and deeply kind. There was warmth in their approach, a sense that they understood the emotional weight behind every medical appointment. They were not just treating bodies; they were helping build families.

One of the most important parts of the journey began at Fertilidad Integral, where from the moment we walked through their doors, we felt reassured. The team at Fertilidad Integral was experienced, supportive, and incredibly thorough. The fertility doctor who led our case walked us through every step, from medication protocols to fertilization techniques, with patience and clarity.

For the first time in this long journey, we were not being rushed or dismissed. We were part of the process.

Around the same time, we were finalizing our egg donor through Her Helping Habit in Vancouver. We spent days going through catalogues of potential donors—reading profiles, studying photos, and learning about each woman's reasons for donating. It was emotional and overwhelming. Every face represented a future. We kept returning to one donor in particular. She had a warm smile with a kind of quiet confidence and gentleness that stood out to us right away. There was something about her that felt deeply aligned with who we were.

Before we went to Mexico City, we arranged to meet her online. Since Her Helping Habit was a known donor agency, this meeting was an important part of the process for all of us. We were nervous, but once the conversation began the nerves melted away. What we expected to be a short, formal call turned into over an hour of connection. We talked openly about life, values, and why we were all on this journey. There was an instant, unexpected bond, a natural ease that reassured us even more that she was the right person. Choosing her did not feel like a transaction. It felt like trusting someone with part of our hearts.

Her decision to be a known donor gave us peace to know we would not have to keep this part of our child's story hidden. They would have the choice, someday, to know where they came from and we would be able to tell them, with full hearts, just how much love and thought went into them from the very beginning.

Then it was time for one of the most surreal and emotional parts of the journey: meeting our surrogate. However, in our case, it did not happen the usual way.

In April of 2022, my husband traveled to Mexico City alone to complete his part of the medical process. At the time, I was a full time teacher and this trip fell in the middle of the school year, but I was able to join virtually.

While in Mexico, Koen met with our coordinator from Gestacy; a warm and thoughtful woman named Bety. I joined the conversation via FaceTime, and from the moment we started talking, we both felt an instant connection. Bety was warm, kind and genuine. It felt more like catching up with someone we already knew than meeting someone for the first time. At the end of the call, Bety said something that caught our attention: she shared that she hoped to become a surrogate one day.

We thought it was a beautiful sentiment, something generous and full of heart. We never imagined it had anything to do with us, but the very next day, I received an email from the owner of Gestacy. He told us that after our conversation, Bety felt so moved by our story and expressed a desire to be our surrogate.

I was completely stunned. That had never happened before. In most cases, intended parents are matched with surrogates through formal, structured steps and it can take a few months for the match to happen. This felt completely organic, unplanned, and somehow, perfectly right. We were in awe of her generosity, of her trust, of her willingness to carry someone else's dream so that we could become parents.

We started a WhatsApp group right away, just the three of us: my husband, Bety, and I. It became our little lifeline, a space where we could stay connected across borders and time zones. We would send each other updates, photos, questions, emojis; sometimes serious, sometimes silly. It was not just about appointments or logistics. It was about a relationship. The beginnings of a partnership built on trust, gratitude, and love.

Around the same time, another critical part of our journey was unfolding. Our egg donor completed her egg retrieval in April of 2022, the very same time Koen was in Mexico City doing his part. Everything was aligned. Our doctor from Fertilidad Integral performed the procedure, and we were overjoyed to learn that he was able to retrieve forty-two eggs, the same number as was our waitlist for adoption. Of those, thirty-four were fertilized, and from that, we ended up with fourteen Day-6 embryos. Our doctor then recommended PGT-A testing for ten of the embryos to assess their chromosomal health. The result? Eight excellent euploid embryos!

For the first time, we had not just hope, but numbers. Tangible, scientific progress. It was a surreal combination of high-tech science and high-stakes emotion, and we were filled with cautious optimism.

We were in awe of our egg donor's generosity, of her trust, of her willingness to carry someone else's dream so that we could become parents.

Over time, a bond began to form. Not one of friendship yet; more like quiet respect and deep gratitude at first. We were strangers brought together by something much larger than ourselves. With the embryo transfer ahead, we started working on legal preparations and medical schedules. There were forms to sign, tests to take, protocols to follow. And yet, underneath all of it, there was a sense of stillness. We were doing this. It was really happening. For the first time in a long time, the waiting had a direction. For the first time in a long time, we were no longer stuck in limbo. We were building a team, and piece by piece, that team was building our family.

CHAPTER 4
The Transfer

Embryo transfer day felt like the quietest kind of miracle, but we did not arrive at that day quickly. Before we could proceed with the transfer, we had to wait eight long months for the legal paperwork to be finalized. That waiting period was agonizing, especially because everything else was ready. The embryos were created, Bety was committed, we were emotionally prepared. However, the legal process stalled.

Our first legal team, whom we had placed our trust in, stopped communicating with us. Emails went unanswered. Timelines drifted. We felt helpless, stuck in limbo with no clear path forward. After months of silence and mounting frustration, we made the difficult decision to fire them and hire a new legal team. It was not a move we made lightly, but this was our family we were trying to build, and time felt both precious and painfully slow.

The new team picked things up quickly, but by that point, valuable months had been lost. Looking back, those eight months were some of the hardest. We had everything in place, the science, the support, the people, and yet we could not move. It was like standing on the threshold of your dream with the door locked from the inside.

So when the day of the transfer finally came on January 13, 2023, it was not just a medical procedure, it was a victory. Bety was calm and ready. She had followed all of the instructions, taken the medications exactly as directed, and shown up with a full heart. We could not be in Mexico City for the transfer in person, which broke my heart a little, but we were there in every other way, texting constantly, sending encouragement, praying.

Our doctor from Fertilidad Integral carefully selected the best embryo from our eight healthy euploid embryos and transferred it into Bety. The transfer went smoothly. The clinic team sent us photos of the embryo; a female, under the microscope, tiny, fragile, and perfect. It was surreal to think: This could be her. Our daughter.

The wait that followed was excruciating. Even though we knew it would be at least ten days before we would get news, we hung on every update, every message from Bety, every feeling she shared. During this time, our WhatsApp group became a lifeline again. Bety told us she was resting, that she felt good. She even ate the McDonald's fries that people tend to do after a transfer for good luck. She sent sweet emojis and little updates that filled our hearts with both joy and anxiety. We were grateful beyond words but also scared to believe this might finally be working.

Then, one day, the message came. Bety asked us if we wanted her to take an at-home pregnancy test. We said yes, of course! Our hearts were racing. She did the test and then asked us, so sweetly, "Do you want to see the results?" We were so nervous. It felt like everything was hanging in that moment, years of hoping and heartbreak, condensed into one plastic stick and a quiet question on WhatsApp.

Then, there it was. A photo of the pregnancy test. Positive! Wrapped in her daughter's favorite toy. I stared at the screen, breathless. A second line. A positive! I remember zooming in on it, staring at it like it was a message from the universe. That little toy astronaut holding the test, so full of innocence, sweetness and life, it undid me. After everything we had been through, this moment cracked something open in me. I cried. Koen cried. We held each other in a quiet, stunned happiness that neither of us had dared let ourselves imagine.

CHAPTER 5
Across Borders

Pregnancy, for most people, is about what's happening inside their body. For us, it was about what was happening across borders, across screens, and inside someone else's heart. After the positive test, our world shifted. We had been holding our breath for years. Now we were breathing, but very carefully. The pregnancy was real. Confirmed. Our daughter was growing inside Bety, in Mexico City, while we remained in Calgary, thousands of kilometers and an entire life away.

Every day, Bety would send us updates. She told us what she was craving, how she was feeling, what the doctors were saying. Sometimes it was clinical, appointments, medications, measurements. Other times it was personal, when she felt tired, when she experienced her first little wave of nausea.

The WhatsApp group became a constant thread in our lives. We checked our phones obsessively. We wanted to be present, even if we could not physically be there. When the first ultrasound came at six weeks and we saw that tiny flickering heartbeat, something shifted in me. I was terrified to fall in love, but there it was, this little light, pulsing with life, refusing to be ignored. We watched the pregnancy unfold in pictures and messages: a tiny growing belly, doctor reports in Spanish that Bety lovingly translated for us, and audio recordings of the heartbeat.

At times, I felt a strange mix of gratitude and grief. I was overwhelmed with thankfulness for Bety, for her care, her strength, her updates, her kindness. And at the same time, I mourned that I was not the one carrying this child. I could not feel the kicks, or lie in bed with a hand on my belly. I could not experience any of it physically. However, emotionally? I felt everything. I lived for the milestones. The 12-week mark, when we could finally exhale just a little. The 20-week anatomy scan, when we saw her profile and little legs. The photos of Bety smiling, her hand resting over the baby, our baby.

In March of 2023, we shared the news with the world. We made a pregnancy and gender announcement on social media with a photo, our baby girl was on her way. It felt surreal to write those words, to finally say it out loud. We told our families and friends personally. There were happy tears and overwhelming joy. After years of holding this dream close, of keeping so much private and sacred, it felt like we were finally stepping into the light. There was still a part of me that held my breath, but there was also a part of me that was ready to believe.

As the months passed, our relationship with Bety deepened. She sent messages that made us laugh. She shared moments with her daughter, who began to understand that her mommy was helping another family grow. There was something powerful about the simplicity of it. Love, carrying love.

In April of 2023, when Bety was about 16 weeks pregnant, we flew down to Mexico City to visit in person. It was a week I will never forget, a chance to truly feel part of the experience, not just witness it through a screen. We spent time with Bety and her family, went to her partner's football game, played with her daughter, and shared meals together at their coffee shop. Everything felt natural, like we were not just intended parents and a surrogate, but people who genuinely cared about one another. It was not clinical. It was personal. That week was full of moments that felt like pure magic.

We also had the chance to meet our egg donor in person, along with her boyfriend. We shared a beautiful dinner with them, full of conversation, warmth, and gratitude. It meant the world to us to connect face to face. Sitting across the table from the woman who had helped make our daughter possible was surreal, emotional, and deeply grounding.

The most unforgettable of all, we got to see our baby in a 3D ultrasound. Bety was glowing. And there she was, our daughter, still growing inside her; her tiny face already taking shape. I remember staring at the screen, unable to speak. We saw her profile, her nose, her little fists tucked beneath her chin. She looked so real.

That visit changed everything. It took something that had felt distant, surreal, and made it tangible. It gave us memories, not just of the process, but of people. It reminded us that this was not just a medical journey. It was a human one. A deeply relational, soul-stretching, heart-expanding experience.

The pregnancy was not without worry. We still feared what might go wrong. We had appointments translated over text, delays in lab reports, and stretches of silence that made our hearts race, but each time we heard that heartbeat, each time we saw her little spine curled into view on a blurry screen, the fear eased. We were becoming parents. Even if the road looked nothing like we imagined.

CHAPTER 6
Preparing for Her

There is a quiet urgency that comes with preparing for a baby you are not carrying yourself. We were not timing contractions or packing a hospital bag. We were booking flights, filling out legal forms, researching newborn passport requirements. Watching the weeks tick by while staring at a calendar and a map. As Bety's belly grew, so did the reality that this was really happening. We were having a baby. In Mexico City. We had to be ready, not just emotionally, but legally, logistically and practically.

There were contracts to finalize, parental recognition documents to arrange, and plans to make for our stay in Mexico City. We did not know exactly when the baby would arrive, but we had to be ready to leave on short notice.

Our lawyer walked us through the legal process for Canadian intended parents giving birth via surrogacy in Mexico. There were forms, translations, court filings, notarizations. It was overwhelming—but also strangely empowering. Every document signed was another step toward becoming her parents on paper, even though we had felt it in our hearts for years.

During this time, our legal team informed us that we would need to stay in Mexico City for two to three months after the birth in order to finalize the legal process and obtain all necessary documentation, including our daughter's passport. We were okay with that. We understood that this was part of the journey, and we started planning for it. Koen would be able to work remotely, which gave us the flexibility we needed. We researched temporary housing, figured out finances, and began to picture what life might look like in Mexico City as new parents, navigating both diapers and immigration paperwork at the same time.

At home in Calgary, we began to nest, even from a distance. We set up the nursery, ordered baby gear and washed tiny clothes and folded them with trembling hands. There was something healing about these small acts, like claiming the space that had once felt so out of reach.

I also did something quiet but deeply meaningful: I bought a small wooden name disc engraved with our daughter's name. I kept it close, on my bedside table, sometimes under my pillow. Each night before I went to sleep, I would hold it in my hands and say a mantra, praying for both Bety and our unborn daughter. *Amalia is safe, Amalia is healthy and growing. Bety is safe, Bety is healthy.* It became a sacred ritual, my way of mothering from afar.

We also started preparing emotionally, for a whole new kind of uncertainty. What would the birth be like? How would it feel to hold her for the first time after so many years of waiting? The tension between excitement and fear was constant, but more than anything, we felt ready. Not in the way that checklists make you ready, but in the way that comes after heartbreak, healing and hope. We had waited long enough. Our daughter was on her way.

At the end of August 2023, something truly special happened - my baby shower. After everything we had been through, to be celebrated like this, surrounded by people who loved us and who had walked this path with us, it felt surreal. My friends hosted it in a beautiful space, filled with laughter, soft colors, and joy. My mother and sister came, which meant the world to me, and my mother-in-law flew all the way from Holland just to be there. It was a room full of love and anticipation and then, on the screen, Bety joined via FaceTime. Seeing her face light up, hearing her voice from across the world, made the day feel complete. Even though she was thousands of kilometers away, her presence was right there in the room with us. It was a magical day, the kind that reminds you just how much love this little girl was already bringing into the world.

CHAPTER 7

The Birth

We always knew the birth would come with uncertainty, flights, timing, nerves, but once the delivery date was set, everything felt suddenly real. Our doctor told us that Bety would have a scheduled C-section on September 15, 2023. So on August 29, 2023, we flew down to Mexico City, suitcases full of baby clothes, documents and hope. We were nervous, excited and full of emotion. We knew we would be waiting about two weeks, but we were grateful for the chance to be close. We did not want to miss a thing.

During those weeks, we went to medical appointments with Bety, checked in with the doctors and followed our daughter's growth closely. We also bought baby items locally, clothes, blankets, bottles, tiny things that made it feel more and more real.

We visited pharmacies and baby stores, choosing each item with a mix of joy and disbelief. This was really happening. We also met with our legal team to finalize the last of the paperwork. Parentage documents, translations, court submissions; it was still a process, but now it felt purposeful. Each signature, each step, brought us closer to holding our daughter in our arms.

As the date approached, every ping from our phones made our hearts race. Bety was doing beautifully, strong, healthy, calm, but we were still bracing ourselves.

Then the morning of September 15, 2023 came, the day we would meet our daughter. We drove to the hospital with

Bety and her partner, Jesús. There was something quiet and sacred about that car ride, no one saying too much, everyone holding a different kind of emotion.

When we arrived, we met our Gestacy coordinator at the hospital entrance. She helped us settle into the room while Bety began getting prepped for her surgery. It was all happening. We were like flies on the wall, watching and listening. Observing every moment, every nurse's instruction, every quiet exchange between Bety and Jesús. We wanted to respect their space, but we also wanted to hold space for what this moment meant.

I remember how Bety was so calm and centered. I do not know how else to describe it. She was so composed, so full of grace. Everything moved quickly, and yet I remember every second. Then, Bety was wheeled into the delivery room, with Jesús following behind her. Koen and I stayed in the room. It was quiet except for the background noise of the TV, where the President of Mexico was giving a speech to the nation. It was Mexican Independence Day - the moment our daughter would be born. We sat in silence, eyes locked, hands clasped. The sound of history playing in the background, the hum of distant footsteps, the buzz of emotion between us. We waited for what felt like an eternity. Time slowed, stretched. We just stared at each other, too full to speak, too overwhelmed to move.

Then suddenly, a ping on my phone. It was a message from Jesús. *"Felicidad, todo bien." Joy. Everything is good.* I exhaled for the first time in what felt like hours. The message was simple, but it carried the weight of everything. Our daughter was here. Safe. Born into a moment larger than all of us. Then came the photos and videos. We saw her, tiny, crying, alive. Her first moments. Her voice. She was here! She was safe! The tears came freely then. Koen and I held each other, crying and laughing and whispering her name over and over.

Shortly after, our doctor came to check on us, smiling with

that calm reassurance we needed so badly. "Amalia and Bety are both doing very well," he said. I felt something inside me soften, release. The years of tension, of trying to hold it all together, began to melt away. We had made it. Our daughter was here and she was okay.

That night, Amalia went for tests, as is common for newborns in Mexico. It was standard procedure, but it meant we wouldn't get to hold her until morning. We went back to our place to try to sleep, but I couldn't. I lay there, heart racing, watching the clock, thinking about her tiny face and the sound of her cry. I was exhausted, but wide awake. I was a mother now and in just a few hours, I would finally get to hold my daughter in my arms.

CHAPTER 8
Becoming Her Mother

The next morning, we rushed to the hospital before the sun came up. I had not slept. My heart had been racing all night, replaying her cry, staring at the ceiling, whispering her name, and then there she was. Amalia. Wrapped in a tiny pink blanket, eyes blinking slowly, impossibly small. Resting in a bassinet next to Bety. The nurse placed her in my arms, and the world just disappeared.

I had imagined that moment for years, through infertility, through therapy, through hope and heartbreak and paperwork, but the reality of it was something else entirely. She was warm. She had a smell and her breath puffed softly against my chest, as I could feel my entire nervous system calm. Koen stood beside me, staring at us. I saw the tears in his eyes before I felt my own. We were finally a family.

The nurses came and went, checking vitals, giving instructions in soft voices. The room was a blur. We spent those first few days in the hospital. We held her every moment we could. We fed her and watched her sleep. We took turns just staring at her face. One of the most unexpected gifts came from Jesús. He gently showed me how to hold her, how to change her diaper, and how to feed her. There was no ego, no awkwardness, just kindness. Just one parent helping another become one.

I had never changed a newborn before and here was Jesús, who had supported Bety through her two pregnancies, offering his quiet expertise with gentleness and respect. It reminded me that this story was about people choosing to care for and help one another. There were moments of awe, and moments of complete overwhelm.

It felt surreal to be doing all of this in Mexico City, where everything was familiar and foreign at the same time. We learned to navigate newborn care and Spanish paperwork in the same breath.

Gestacy, our coordinator, our doctor and the nurses were incredible. They guided us, translated, and reassured us. And Bety, gracious and strong, was resting and recovering. We texted often, sent photos, and stayed connected as Amalia's life began.

Koen was finally a father and as he sang softly to her in Dutch, the three of us fell asleep in the room together for the very first time. We were exhausted and completely full. I was a mother and Koen was a father. Not just in name, not just in hope, but in practice, in presence, in love.

CHAPTER 9
In Limbo

Amalia came home with us, and everything changed. Our little apartment transformed into a haven of burp cloths, tiny clothes, baby cries, and wonder. The city outside bustled with color and chaos, but inside, our world had narrowed to the weight of one tiny life.

We had the blessing of Koen's mother staying with us during those early weeks. She helped us settle in, cooked for us, and filled our space with comfort and care. Her presence allowed us to rest, to focus, to breathe. Soon after, Koen's father came to meet Amalia, making the journey from Holland to hold his granddaughter. After a precious week together, he returned home to the Netherlands with Koen's mother, and then, one by one, more family arrived. My sister-in-law and niece came next, filling the space with laughter and warmth. Then, my mother came to be by our side. It was incredibly moving to watch each person meet Amalia for the first time. There was so much awe, so many quiet tears. After all the years of hoping and waiting, it felt like the world was finally catching up to the dream that had lived in our hearts for so long.

We were learning everything from scratch. How to bathe a slippery newborn. How to swaddle just right. How to soothe her cries in the middle of the night. We went for slow, stroller-pushing walks through Lincoln Park and Parque América, soaking in the soft warmth of the sun and the shade of the trees. It felt surreal, becoming parents in such a vibrant, historic city.

However, while our hearts were full, the legal process was still dragging. The lawyers continued to say that everything was pending. Delays piled on delays. What we thought would be a few weeks stretched into months. We were now caught in a federal court battle, trying to have both of us legally recognized as parents on Amalia's birth certificate. It was exhausting. Some days it felt like we were climbing a mountain barefoot. Then one day we looked up and realized it was December. Christmas in Mexico City. We had brought one newborn outfit for Amalia's "first Christmas," never imagining we would still be here. The city sparkled with lights and music, and we tried our best to find joy in the beauty around us, but there was also a quiet ache. We were still in limbo. Still waiting. Unable to go home.

So, we made a decision. We reached out to other intended parents who were also stuck in Mexico City, waiting on legal outcomes just like us, and we invited them to spend Christmas dinner with us. It was not the holiday we had imagined, but it became something truly special. We shared food, stories, and laughter. We passed babies from one arm to the next. We found comfort in each other's presence, all of us strangers who had suddenly become family by circumstance.

Unfortunately the legal tension loomed and then, everything took a turn for the worse. One day, we got the news that the judge had decided not to put my name on Amalia's birth certificate. I remember reading that sentence and feeling like the air had been sucked out of the room. After everything we had been through, I was being told, on paper, that I did not exist in my own daughter's life. We had to go down to the court ourselves to fight it. It was tense, humiliating, and deeply personal. We had to plead our case again for the right to be recognized as Amalia's mother. After more months, we eventually won, and my name was added. However, the emotional damage had been done. It traumatized me. To feel so powerless in a moment that should have been about family and love, left me with scars. I smiled for Amalia, I stayed strong for Koen, but inside I felt like I was unraveling. Surrogacy had brought us the greatest joy of our lives, but the bureaucratic system around it had also exposed us to some of our deepest pain. It would not be until early March of 2024 that we were finally allowed to come home.

CHAPTER 10
Coming Home

After everything, the hospital, the paperwork, the courtrooms, the joy, the trauma, we finally heard the words we had been longing for:

"You can go home. Here is your daughter's passport".

It was early March, nearly six months after Amalia's birth.

We packed our bags with disbelief. The same ones we had brought down in August, filled with tiny baby clothes and one hopeful Christmas outfit, were now stuffed with diapers, documents, and memories we had not known we would make. Mexico City had become a part of us. As we said goodbye to our apartment, the parks, the people, and the city that had held our most sacred chapter, I felt a deep ache, as well as gratitude, exhaustion and of course, love.

We said goodbye to our friends, the ones who had become our surrogate family during this journey and most tenderly, we said goodbye to our amazing surrogate, Bety, and to our incredible egg donor. There were hugs and tears, quiet words of thanks, and long moments of simply holding each other. We promised to stay in touch. We promised to never forget. It was so bittersweet. We were finally going home as a family of three.

EPILOGUE
Love Always Finds A Way

I sit in Amalia's room, watching her sleep, soft breaths with her small fingers curled around my hand. Sometimes I still cannot believe she is real, that she is mine. After everything - the diagnoses, the delays, the plane rides, the courtrooms, the heartbreak- she is finally here.

Mexico City lives inside of us now. In the scent of strong coffee, in the trees of Lincoln Park, in the flavor of the chilaquiles, in WhatsApp messages with Bety, and in the quiet memory of that moment we first heard her cry. I think of Bety often, her courage, her kindness, the sacred gift she gave. I think of our egg donor, whose generosity began it all. I think of the others we met along the way, parents waiting, families forming in the middle of uncertainty. I think of the woman I used to be, the one who started this journey unsure, heartbroken, hopeful.

To her I would like to say:

Keep going. Never give up. Love always finds a way.

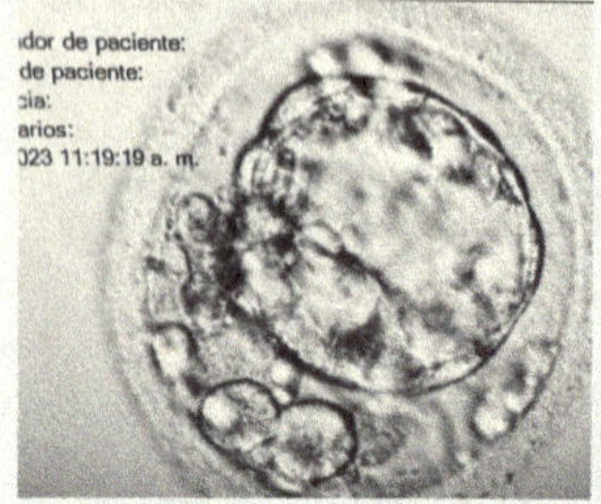

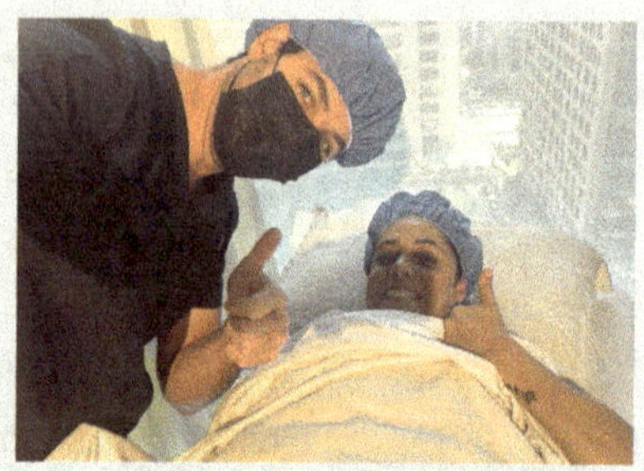

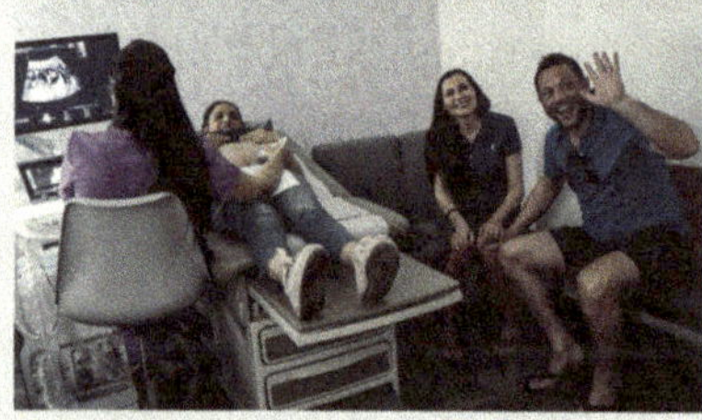

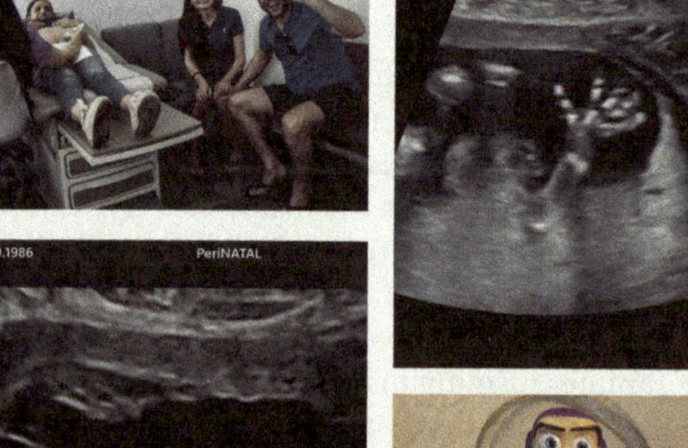

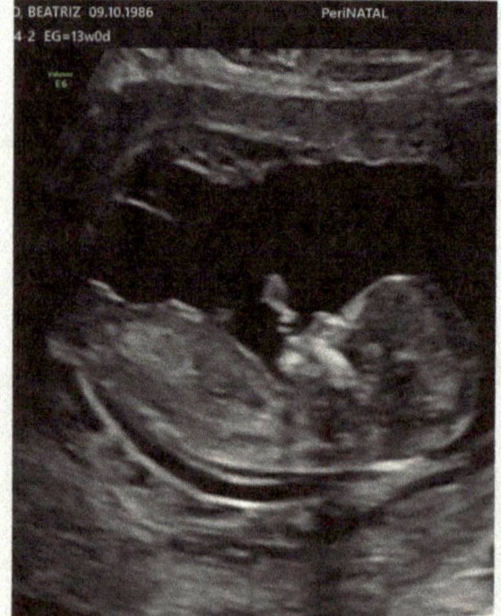

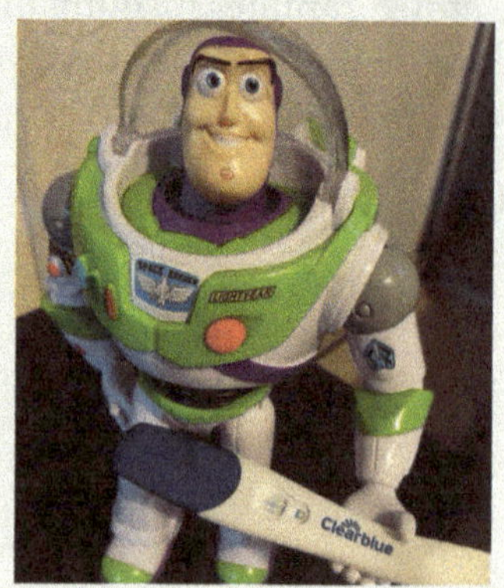

Where Hope Took Root ♥

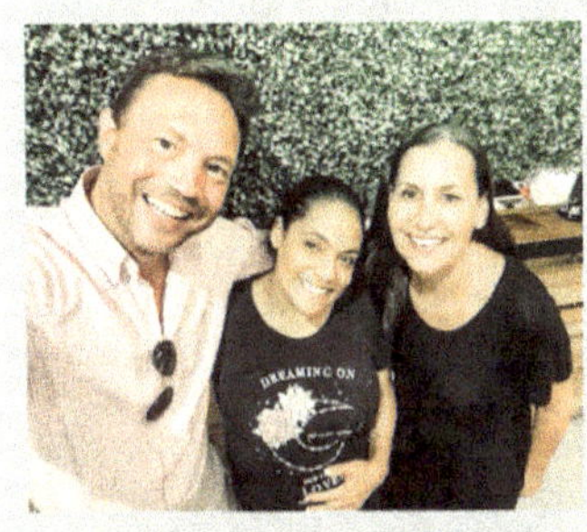

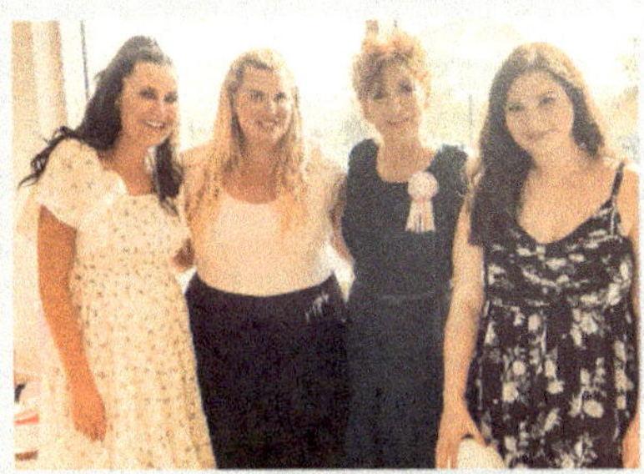

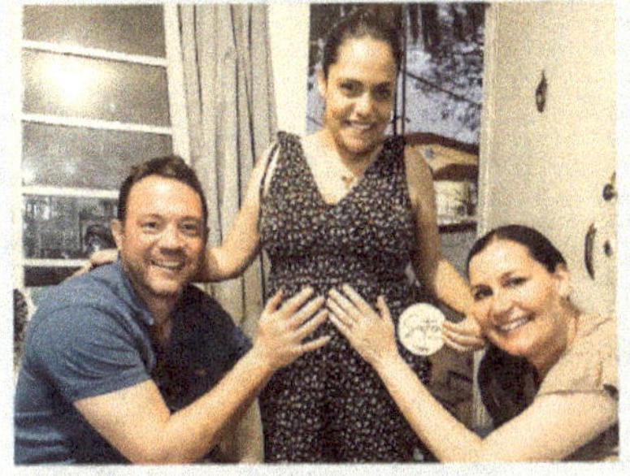

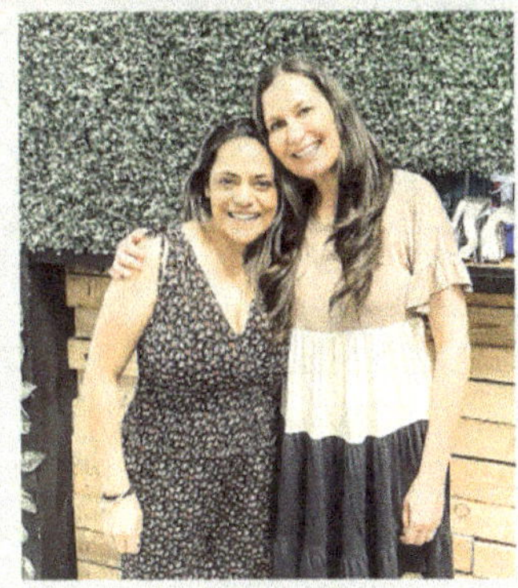

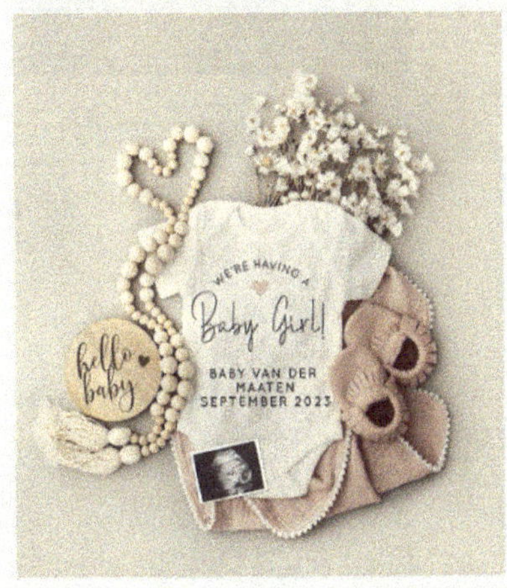

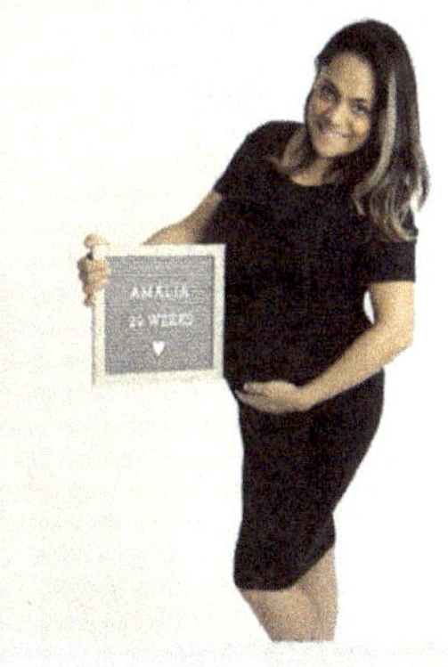

Carried With Love ♥

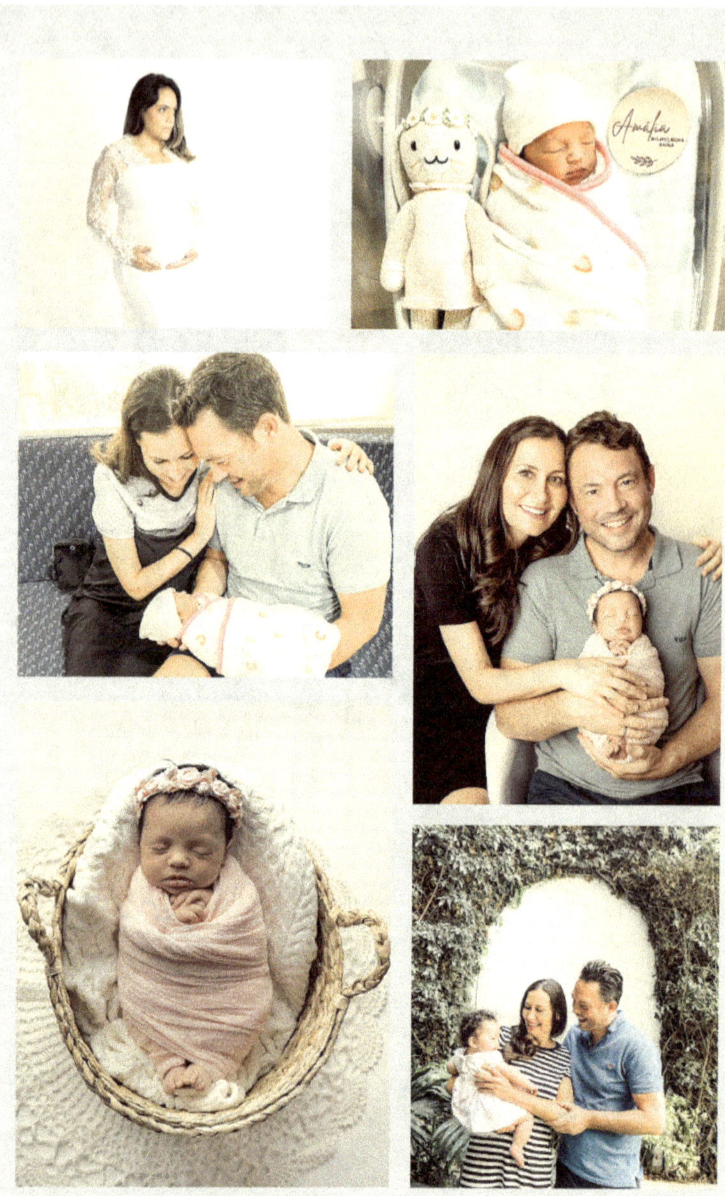

Born From The Heart ♥

PART II
Reflections From Those Who Walked With Us

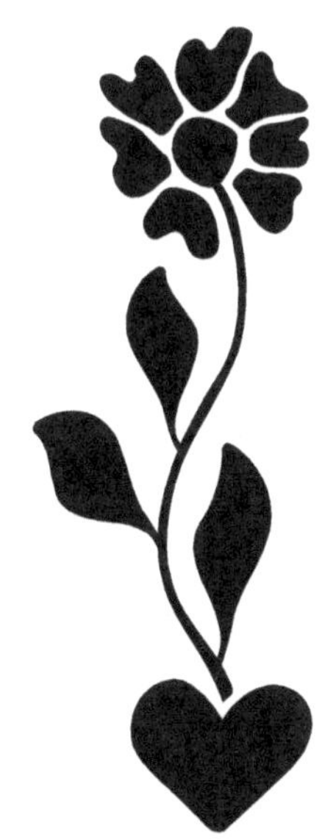

From The Heart of Bety

OUR SURROGATE

I never imagined that something that started with a simple informational call would become one of the most profound and beautiful experiences of my life.

When I first met Barbara and Koen, I was only supposed to explain how surrogacy works in Mexico, but from the very first minutes, I felt something different. There was an instant closeness, the kind you feel when you meet someone and immediately like them, almost as if you had known them before.

Without realizing it, that first exchange full of trust, nervous laughter, and small coincidences began to grow. What started as a conversation between strangers slowly became a genuine friendship, and eventually, a family.

I never thought I would be capable, physically or emotionally, of going through a surrogacy journey. Today, I feel deeply happy, and I can say with certainty that they grew their family, but we grew ours too. We are, with so much pride, a beautiful story to tell, one we will always want to share with the world to inspire hope and give comfort to all the families fighting their own battles out there. Not only against infertility, but also against social challenges, legal barriers, stigma and the absence of accurate information.

As I got to know Barbara and Koen, we discovered something that made me smile inside: we all love music, especially rock. We like the same bands, Guns N' Roses among them and both of our families are full of musicians. So Amalia, who didn't even exist yet, already had a strong musical influence waiting for her.

From that moment, even if I didn't say it out loud, I already saw them as parents. And why wouldn't they be? They had so much love, so much strength, so much desire, that my heart knew something beautiful was about to happen. I felt I had to do more than just explain a process I had to walk with them.

We were incredibly lucky - we only needed one embryo transfer.

The fear of disappointing Barbara and Koen, if it didn't work, was enormous. I carried their dream inside my body, beating almost at the same rhythm as my own heart. Those ten days of beta-wait felt like forever! We took a home pregnancy test too early, and it came back negative (yes, we did it, we knew it was a probability to be negative). We repeated it the day before the beta and there it was - life. Positive! A strong, clear, beautiful positive. I sent them the photo, we cried together on a video call, and the next day came the official confirmation.

After that came the deepest part. Once pregnant, I understood I now had to protect a baby that was not mine, but who lived inside my body. I felt an immense, tender responsibility. I cared for myself more than ever. Every step, every meal, every decision I made then was thinking of protecting that tiny heart. Towards the end of the pregnancy, my body asked me to stop working, so I had to take a break. At the same time, I felt something very strong in my own heart: I wanted to play with my daughter again, to run with her, to hug her. She was only three years old, and even though she understood in her own way, I knew I had to take extra care during that last stretch, for her, for the baby, and for myself. I learned that a surrogate must take great care of herself and make her well-being a priority, but also that the love for your own children continues to guide you and keep you grounded.

But I was so lucky: my intended parents were warm, kind, and deeply respectful. They always protected my space, my privacy, my life. They never crossed a line. They never asked for anything that made me uncomfortable. They always trusted me. And that trust changed everything.

This pregnancy was not like the one with my daughter. It was different, more conscious, more delicate. I shared every ultrasound, every picture, every movement with them. (And oh my God… the heartburn! Haha.) But everything made sense. What I didn't know was that the day Amalia was born, our extended family was born too. Without realizing it, that day, not only did a baby come into the world, a lifelong bond was born. Unknowingly, a safer path for many other families around the world was born as well. That was the moment I understood my story wasn't ending, it was just beginning.

Two years later, watching them live exactly the dream they once described to me is hard to put into words. Knowing I was part of that, that my hands, my body, and my heart helped create that family, fills me with a pride that doesn't fade. The most beautiful part is that we are still family. We write to each other, we visit, we share music, stories, and love. They have come to Mexico; we have lived unforgettable moments, and some sad and difficult moments too. We are planning to visit them in Canada, where we are always welcomed with open arms. This is not just a surrogacy story; it is a story of connection, of love, and of a chosen family.

The most beautiful thing is that I am still on this path. I continue to see families grow and support surrogates with real empathy. I continue to guide parents who need honest information and safe processes. My experience as a surrogate and as a coordinator gave me a wide, human, and necessary perspective, one I felt I needed to share. Above all, I am happy to have them in my life. Without a doubt,

Amalia has golden parents and I wish her to have a life full of happiness and, above all, a lot of love!

I am happy that our story didn't end at birth, but instead opened a new extended family. I'm excited to see what other adventures, surprises, and beautiful moments life has in store for us and new surrogacy friends around the world! This bond is so unique and ours is just beginning. Surrogacy has something truly wonderful: here, the search ends. Here, you will become a mom or a dad. Without a doubt.

That is why, when a family reaches out to me, to me... they are already parents. We are simply waiting for their story to reach the chapter where they finally get to hold their baby.

From the Heart of Dr Frusch

OUR REPRODUCTIVE ENDOCRINOLOGIST

Life as a reproductive endocrinologist is not always easy. As we see patients come and go, it is easy to lose sight of what is truly important. It isn't that we don't care or lack the desire to help, but—much like biological systems that become desensitized to constant stimuli—we can become desensitized over time. This is a natural defense mechanism, yet it risks normalizing a process that, for our patients, represents their greatest hope, their deepest dream, and their ultimate objective.

This is why every morning I recall my father's words: *"Always remember that for the patient in front of you, it is their first time."* Whether they are facing the heartbreak of infertility, searching for answers, or experiencing the miracle of birth, I remind myself that even though I have lived this thousands of times, for them, it is a singular, life-changing moment. Whether it is lived through excitement, joy, or sadness, we must never forget that they are navigating a unique and sacred experience.

With this in mind, we must also recognize that we are often tasked with decisions that fall outside the clinical world we were trained in. Many of these choices reside in ethical, moral, and legal gray areas where the pathways are not always clear. It was within this complexity that I had the joy of meeting Barbara and Koen. I have always advocated that as long as we work within the legal and ethical frameworks of a country, we should do everything in our power to help couples fulfill their dreams of forming a family.

I will not dwell on the many complexities of the legal and bureaucratic framework in Mexico—which I am certain will be detailed elsewhere in this book—but I must share what a pleasure it was to find, on the other side of the screen, a couple so genuinely excited. I remember hanging up after our first online visit; my fertility coordinator, who was still learning the intricacies of our field, looked at me with wide eyes, eager to understand how a surrogacy journey actually works. I simply smiled. I knew it would be a challenge to get a young team up to speed on the SOPs, legal requirements, donor coordination, and psychological screenings. However, the excitement of helping a couple who had endured so much, along with the joy of seeing the smiles on Barbara and Koen's faces when we told them we could help — and on a timeline they never anticipated — made it all worthwhile.

I will leave the specific details of their journey to Barbara and Koen, as no one can tell their story better than they can. But I will say this: as a physician, surrogacy is often surrounded by controversy. It carries a social, legal, and human complexity that forces us to question the best path forward every day. Unfortunately, there are stories that make us fear that science is moving too fast, or that the line between what we *can* do and what we *should* do has blurred.

Barbara and Koen, in conjunction with the Gestacy team, showed us exactly how it should be done. They approached the process with clear intention, exhaustive research, and a deep appreciation for their surrogate, whom they embraced as part of their family. They crossed every "t" and dotted every "i" to ensure the process was safe, transparent, and ethical. By doing so, they have created a pathway for others to follow. They are sharing their story knowing they may face both applause and criticism, but they do so to increase accessibility for other families. They are advocates for ethical pathways where surrogates are protected and honored for the beautiful sacrifice they make.

What I saw from our first meeting — and what remained true throughout their treatment — was a couple who desperately wanted a family but refused to take shortcuts that would compromise the integrity of the process or the well-being of anyone involved. They faced their share of hardships, but they stayed with a course defined by transparency and integrity. Above all, I am so happy to have met Amália. The best payment we get is the picture of the family after we have done the best job we can. It doesn't matter where you practice reproductive medicine, we all agree, and even though it's the millionth time we get a picture we always smile.

I am grateful and humbled to have been allowed to play a part in this journey.

With great affection,

Dr. José Gutiérrez Frusch

From the Heart of Koen

HUSBAND & FATHER

Growing up in a relatively small family with only one sister and a handful of cousins, I always wanted a busy household of my own. I loved the idea of a dinner table packed full of kids, laughing, joking around, being mischievous, with me as a father, quietly observing at the head of the table.

As so often happens though, life turned out a bit differently. In my early thirties, I moved from the Netherlands to Canada for a business opportunity. It was there that I met my wife Barbara. We fell in love and married within a year of meeting each other.

I was 33 at the time and Barbara was 29. We had married quickly and still wanted a lot of time to explore each other as a married couple. On top of that, my business in Canada was still young and Babara just started her teaching career, so the immediate urge to start a family was not there.

Barbara and I travelled a lot, got to know each other even better, my business became more mature, and after approximately 5 years of marriage, we really wanted to start a family. Barbara was around 34 at that time. While perhaps a bit older than average to start a family, there was no history in her family of any fertility issues whatsoever, so we really didn't think that we would encounter any problems having children.

However, going about it in the old-fashioned way yielded no results. So, after about a year of trying we went to a fertility clinic. They performed tests on both of us, and we learned that Barbara had diminished ovarian reserves. In addition, she had many cysts and fibroids as well as endometriosis, creating a rather inhospitable environment. The doctor was quick to point out that IVF would be of no use at all, and completing a pregnancy was also highly unlikely.

Apart from being appalled by the horrible bedside manner of the doctor, I was rather numb in my initial reaction to the news. Men are not meant to carry babies in a womb; we do not give birth or breastfeed. The act of procreation is typically a fun-filled adventure in the bedroom, and that is about as much as we can contribute. My brain just instantly reverted to coming up with solutions.

For Barbara of course, the news hit a lot harder. As soon as we left the hospital, she burst into tears. Not only was she confronted with the certainty of a genetic loss if we were to have a child, but she also was told that she would not be able to be pregnant - ever. Over the years, I have tried to imagine what she must have felt like on that day, and the many days and years of struggle that followed. To this day, I find it very difficult to think about. I decided that the best I can do is to just listen and be there for her when she is having a rough moment.

It always seemed tremendously unfair to me. Barbara is a Kindergarten Teacher. She has an absolutely amazing way of interacting with little kids. I loved coming into her classroom and seeing all these boys and girls just absolutely adoring her.

Many of Barbara's colleagues have children, and we became close with some of them. We would take some of their kids out to the movies, go out for dinners and even do sleepovers. While amazingly fun, it obviously cannot compare to having your own children.

I know that life is unfair to many people, but it certainly

seemed harsh to me that someone so talented with teaching - and often partially raising - other people's children, would not have any of her own.

After taking some time to process the news, we slowly started thinking of alternative ways to have a family. What so many people take for granted as a simple and fun way to have children, for us became an analysis of finances, time, many hours of research, and ultimately weighing many options.

Our initial approach was to create a family via adoption. International adoption was our first preference. There is something beautiful and almost romantic about travelling to a very foreign country and culture, rescuing a cute little boy or girl from an orphanage, bringing them home and living happily ever after. The reality is very different, however. It involves almost endless amounts of paperwork, home-studies and dealing with numerous different agencies, only to have government interference with closing borders on a country and needing to start all over again.

The international route seems almost like an impossible dream. Especially when you are getting a bit older and time is starting to play a factor. We then switched our approach to domestic adoption. In Alberta, Canada, where we live, this is by law an open-adoption. What this means is that there is complete open communication between the birth-mother, the intended-parents and ultimately the child. For us, this completely fit with our own philosophy. We always believed in being fully transparent with our child. Many studies have shown that it is much better for the child if they know their history from a young age. However, what never felt right to me was the endless levels of gratitude that we were supposed to radiate towards the potential birth mother.

Perhaps it was our adoption agency pushing this, but this constant reminder of how thankful we should be for receiving this child, felt like an unnatural one-way bias. While obviously grateful for the possibility it would happen, my thoughts always were that we as a couple had a lot to offer this potential baby. In Alberta, as we found out, many babies placed for adoption are from mothers with rather bleak future prospects. Many of them are homeless. The notion that we might be rescuing a child from a life on the streets, or worse, was never mentioned or even acknowledged by any of the social workers or other agency people. We just had to be eternally grateful. It always felt off to me.

After re-doing all our paperwork, home-studies, criminal background checks, we were finally on the domestic adoption waitlist. By this time, Barbara was in her late thirties, and I was well into my forties. We were told that the typical wait-time from this point was 2-3 years.

Then the pandemic hit, and after 4-years on a waitlist, barely edging upwards, we were getting desperate. At the start of 2022 (Barbara 42, me 46), we decided it was time for a change of plans.

Years prior, Barbara had looked into surrogacy and egg-donation. The focus had been on doing the process in Canada. Financially, this was completely out of our league at the time, hence the decision for adoption. In addition, in Canada this process follows a complete altruistic model. You cannot commercially compensate someone for helping you start a family. While this perhaps sounds like the morally correct approach on paper, in reality this system is broken in so many ways that go beyond the scope of my story.

In January 2022, fueled by our disastrous adoption journey, Barbara started looking into surrogacy internationally. She quickly found out that Mexico was actually allowing surrogacy, and also allowing commercial agencies to be involved. I had recently had a bit of a windfall with my business, so financially it seemed feasible this time.

The idea was to create embryos from an egg donor, but with my genetic material, and then transfer the embryo into our surrogate in Mexico City. It seemed like a wild idea to me at first. When I first thought of Mexico City, I was overcome by all the stereotypes. Dangerous, corrupt, bureaucratic. While stereotypes are there for a reason, I have grown to completely love that city.

I was also, while still feeling some guilt, excited by the idea that a potential baby would be genetically mine. With adoption, Barbara and I were on the same genetic level (neither), whereas now, I would have a genetic link to the child. I think I was afraid to really bring up this topic at the start of this journey, not wanting to hurt Barbara. Barbara also didn't really open up on this until later.

There were two major decisions to make: finding an egg-donor and selecting a surrogacy agency. Barbara did all the heavy-lifting in terms of research. It often felt like I was a passenger on this enormous freight-train that was very determined to get to its destination.

Going through the egg-donation selection process feels somewhat like going through an online dating website. You read all these profiles of women, with all their physical characteristics, hobbies, education and more. All that is going through my head is this surreal thought of creating a baby with one of them.

I quickly decided that Barbara should have a lead and certainly the final decision on the selection process. That only seemed fair to me, since she was the one suffering the genetic loss.

We could not really settle on any egg donor in Canada (again, the selection is somewhat limited as the process is fully altruistic). Barbara found an agency, Her Helping Habit, who had an affiliate agency, Travelling Donors, for international egg donors. This opened up a much wider selection of egg donors, and we finally found what seemed to be the perfect candidate.

This is when it started to feel real for me for the first time. An online meeting with her was scheduled, and literally within weeks of our decision to look into surrogacy and egg-donation, we were having an amazing chat with our future egg donor. Barbara and I both fell in love with her personality. When both sides agreed this would be a good fit, contracts were drafted and preparations made. After 7-years of no results in adoption, getting this set up in a matter of weeks felt like lightning speed!

The owner of Travelling Donors was extremely helpful in referring us to two other really important parts of the equation: a surrogacy agency with a program in Mexico City and a fertility clinic. The surrogacy agency was Gestacy and the clinic Fertilidad Integral.

For me, the contrast between our Canadian adoption agency and medical clinics compared to these Mexican counterparts could not have been starker. Gestacy made us feel so warm and welcome. Santiago, one of the co-founders, explained the process to us and gave us so much hope. What I appreciated most about him was his honesty. He was not trying to sell us anything. He was realistic in that there would be 'bumps' along the road, but that the outcome would be one of happiness. He could not have been more accurate.

The experience with Fertilidad Integral (FI) was similar. They were very welcoming, professional and kind. In Canada, we were told that we should have had children in our early twenties. Doctors make you feel guilty and impress on you that your infertility is, in part, your own fault. At FI, Dr. Jose Gutiérrez took ample time to listen to our journey and explain the whole IVF process with our egg-donor.

What we did learn through these meetings is that, while 100% legal in Mexico, the concept of surrogacy is still in its infancy. While I started to feel pretty confident in the whole medical side of our journey, the legal aspect seemed somewhat hazy, to say the least. This gut feeling turned out to be correct.

First and foremost, we needed to create embryos. Even though my sperm was checked, I had simply never caused a pregnancy, so I was still somewhat sceptical that 'my guys' would actually be able to do the job. In April 2022, our egg donor was ready to do her retrieval, so it was time for me to fly down to Mexico City so that we could create embryos from freshly retrieved eggs and my sperm. In the months prior, I had given up all alcohol, eaten tons of walnuts (which can be shown to increase sperm count), and wore loose fitting clothes, all in an effort to boost the little soldiers.

I had never visited Mexico City. Flying in at night is the most incredible light show of the city's vastness, with over 20 million people, shows amazingly well that way.

Besides the main event, my visit to Mexico City was also an opportunity to meet our coordinator from Gestacy for the surrogacy journey. Beatriz as I first was introduced to her, Bety as we would come to know her, came to my hotel for a chat. We decided to do FaceTime with Barbara, who was still in Calgary, on the hotel's patio. Bety had a very kind, bubbly, happy type of personality. Chatting with her was so effortless. Barbara and I spoke about us as a couple, how we met, our journey to this point. Bety told us about her family, her daughter and partner. It was a really nice meeting, and in a way, it felt like I had known her already a long time.

At the end of our conversation, Bety mentioned that at some point in her life she would like to be a surrogate for a family herself. I thought it was a nice comment, but she made it so casually at the end, that I honestly did not think too much of it.

The next day however, Barbara received an email from Santiago. He told us that Bety had expressed a desire to be our surrogate. I have to admit that my initial internal reaction was, "did she really think about this enough?" Barbara, who tends to have better judgement of character most times, was over the moon excited. Could it be that within about two months we would have embryos and be matched with a surrogate? Again, this was warp-speed ahead compared to adoption.

More good news happened in the days that followed. On Easter Sunday, I went to Fertilidad Integral. It was the day that our egg-donor would have her 'retrieval' as it is called in medical jargon. I made my way to the clinic. Once there, I handed over my passport to the security officer downstairs and waited by the elevators. It was at the elevators that I met our egg-donor, for the first time. I recognized her from our online meeting and pictures. I called out her name. She seemed a bit startled at first and it felt almost unreal to see her there. We quickly took an awkward selfie in the clinic. We had about 5 minutes to wait, and right away it felt so effortless and nice to chat with her. I asked about how the treatments had been, and we spoke about a few other topics. I think we were both a bit nervous, but it was right away a confirmation that she had been the perfect fit for us.

She was then called into the surgery room and I was guided to one of the deposit rooms. Having done this now a few times for testing purposes, I felt like a pro at this. However, I will always remember thinking that this would be the one which would potentially turn into a son or daughter.

Of the 42 eggs retrieved, 32 were fertilized and in the end we had 10 blastocysts. We had all 10 PGTA tested and 8 came back as healthy embryos. I couldn't believe these amazing results. The 8 healthy embryos were frozen and now it was time for the legal portion of our journey. Our surrogacy contract between us and Bety had to be drafted.

In the months that followed, I had some deja-vu feelings from our adoption days. An enormous amount of paperwork was requested, and everything had to be translated into Spanish as well. From birth certificates to legal guardian statements, utility bills and powers of attorney, t was overwhelming.

In the meantime, our first legal firm in Mexico City (we ended up using 3 different law firms) was not making any progress on the contract. The good old "mañana, mañana" stereotype reared its ugly head—emails went unanswered, timelines slipped, and urgency was repeatedly deferred. After several months without answers or a contract, our agency, Gestacy, decided we should switch legal firms. I remember being afraid we would have to start all the paperwork again, but thankfully, after exerting some pressure, the previous legal firm released all our files.

Finally, on Jan 13, 2023, all the paperwork was signed, Bety was prepped by the amazing FI team and the transfer of one of our embryos happened. It was then that I learned that eating McDonalds French Fries after transfer is a good-luck tradition in the IVF world, so we did.

After all these years with so much paperwork, money spent, and mostly waiting, I was actually remarkably optimistic. I really felt like the first transfer would stick, and indeed, nine days later, Bety took a home pregnancy test. She had the cutest way of telling us that she was pregnant. She put both tests (she did it twice to be sure) on a Toy Story doll and sent the picture to us. To say that it was an amazing feeling would be the understatement of the year.

In the months that followed, my wonder and appreciation for nature took on a whole new level. Hearing the first heartbeat, already after only 6 weeks, is simply astonishing. How do all these cells know what to form?

Modern technology fortunately makes it possible to witness most medical events remotely, but in April of 2023 we went down to Mexico City to be present at one of Bety's ultrasounds. The week that we stayed there was probably one of the most emotional weeks of our lives. Not only did we see our little daughter on the ultrasound screen happily moving and jumping around, we also got to hang out with Bety and her family. We also had an amazing dinner with our egg donor, who Barbara was meeting for the first time, and her boyfriend. Barbara was nervous, almost like she was going on a first date, which I thought was so cute. To this day, she and I really value having this relationship with our egg donor.

Amalia was born on September 15, 2023. The weeks leading up to this were hectic. We were settling into our apartment in Mexico City, we did many more medical checks just prior to birth and had meetings with our coordinator to prepare us for the hospital procedures.

Thankfully my mom had flown in from the Netherlands. First, to Calgary, and then with us to Mexico City. It was really special having her there. My mom would just take care of our food intake, making sure we ate. She became the ridiculously overpriced butcher's new best friend at the local Ingredienta Supermarket.

We had decided that Bety's partner, Jesus, would be present in the delivery room. Barbara and I ended up waiting in Bety's hospital room. September 15th is Mexico's Independence Day, and it is a tradition that the President gives a speech that lasts for hours and hours. We nervously watched the speech on TV, and at around 21:30 I got a text from Jesus: "Felicidades, todos bien". Immediately following this text came a barrage of pictures and videos. An unbelievable feeling. We watched pictures and videos of our beautiful little girl over and over and over again. I remember her ears were a bit crumpled, like rugby player ears. I was thinking that I would love her nonetheless and we would just grow her hair long. Of course this was just the cartilage settling in, and her ears were beautiful the next day.

The next day, after a night of no sleep and just looking at the pictures, we got to meet our daughter for the first time. Holding her felt surreal, almost like she still was not mine and that I would have to give her back any moment. However, Bety was recovering quickly and later that same day she was determined to go back home. Therefore, we got to bring Amalia home with us. I felt that it was rather irresponsible to just give a newborn baby to new parents who have never done this before, without any instruction manual. How were we supposed to take care of this precious little life? Turns out, all parents go through the same fears and we ended up figuring it out.

Our stay in Mexico City ended up lasting six months. This was about double the time we had been told it would take for all the legal logistics to be completed. The main legal step that had to be completed was getting a birth certificate for Amalia naming both Barbara and I as her parents. This is not straightforward in surrogacy cases in Mexico, and has to be accomplished through an Amparo process. Essentially, that is a legal lawsuit from Intended Parents to the Civil Registry, handled by the Federal Family Law courts. For the purpose of my perspective, especially since I got heavily involved in this aspect of our journey, I think this deserves some background.

While surrogacy was legalized by the Supreme Court of Mexico in 2021, the Supreme Court left it up to the individual states of Mexico as to how to implement this right of Assisted Human Reproduction (AHR) via surrogacy.

The issue with this is that all the lower courts, down to the Civil Registry, are either simply refusing to deal with surrogacy, are making it cumbersome, or are including personal bias on surrogacy in their rulings. As a result, your human rights and the rights of your child are violated many times. Having always lived in what are generally considered law-abiding countries, the concept of one court violating the rulings of another - particularly a higher court, is unthinkable.

I can count a total of five times that lower courts violated the Supreme Court ruling in our case.

Violation #1: Our legal journey already started during Bety's pregnancy. Our lawyers at that time presented our case to the Family Court in Mexico City. That presentation included, among many other documents, a fully-executed legal surrogacy agreement that clearly outlined our Procreational Will and also clearly stated that Bety had no intention of being a mother to our baby. In accordance with the Supreme Court ruling, this presentation should have ensured that Barbara and I would be recognized as the parents of Amalia from the moment she was born. However, the Family Court judge simply decided that she did not want to deal with surrogacy and therefore dismissed the case, saying it didn't belong in her court room.

Violation #2: We then (still during pregnancy) appealed this judge's decision with the Magistrates (supervisors – three of them) of this Family Court. The appeal stated that surrogacy, and the recognition of Barbara and I as legal parents, clearly is a matter of the Family Court and that the judge should see our case. The Magistrates ruled 2-1 against our appeal.

Violation #3: With no appeal left to deal with this pre-birth, we now had to wait until Amalia was born. After birth, we would try and get her registered at the Civil Registry with Barbara and I as parents. We went on September 18th with all paperwork, including the surrogacy agreement, to the Central Civil Registry. These civil registries also have "judges." I believe they are the very lowest in the hierarchy, but they are still considered judges. The civil registry also denied the registration of Amalia, essentially stating that they do not have an internal framework to deal with surrogacy. This argument is completely flawed, of course, as they should simply follow the rule of law and issue a birth certificate right away like for any other couple trying to register their child, but this is Mexico.

Violation #4: The next step is to file the beforementioned Amparo. This is a federal injunction against the Civil Registry. Essentially, we had to sue the Civil Registry for not issuing the birth certificate for Amalia. Amparos deal with any constitutional injustices and this is clearly one of them. The Amparo filing again includes all documentation regarding the surrogacy, including the surrogacy agreement.

The entire Amparo process was handled by Leon Altamirano, our third lawyer. He runs a law firm called Altamirano Law and he has tremendous experience in Surrogacy Law, because it's all he does. He is from Tabasco originally, and was part of getting that 2021 ruling from the Supreme Court.

The federal court in Mexico City is made up of 15 courts, each with their own judge. You have no control over which court will handle your case. It gets randomly assigned when you file the Amparo. Personal bias is huge here. Some judges will be surrogacy "friendly" and others not so much. We ended up in Court #4 and our judge turned out to be not very friendly.

Amparos can take quite long to resolve (at least several months). This is why, in order to protect the rights of the newborn child, typically a birth certificate is issued right away upon filing the Amparo. This birth certificate has the legal status of "Provisional." It should allow you to get the child basic essential rights and services like healthcare, but the birth certificate is not "Definitive" until the judge provides his or her final judgement on the Amparo.

In our case, the judge decided that he did not even want to issue even a Provisional birth certificate. He had a really absurd argument that it would violate his legal rights as a judge. He ruled that it was his right to do a thorough review of the case and make changes to the birth certificate if deemed necessary depending on his review. What is even more strange is that our lawyer had filed an identical Amparo with him about a month prior (for two gay dads) and he did issue the Provisional birth certificate then. I thus considered this violation #4.

Violation #5: We then appealed this judge's decision to not issue the Provisional birth certificate with the Federal Court Magistrates (again three of them, supervision the federal court judges in this case). The Magistrates reviewed our case and then made an even more strange decision; they ruled (unanimously) and told the judge that:

a) Yes, a provisional birth certificate should be issued right away to protect the best interest of the child, but,

b) That only I (Koen) and not Barbara should be listed as parents on the birth certificate. Barbara's legal

> parentage status could not be determined yet, until such time that the case was more thoroughly reviewed. My (Koen) parentage was established due to a DNA test that was included in the documentation.

This is a massive violation of the AHR surrogacy ruling of the Supreme Court. Violation #5. The Supreme Court was very clear on the issue of Procreational Will and that parentage has nothing to do with DNA.

Additionally, there is another law in Mexico that states that "any child born into a marriage is automatically a child of both parents". The fact that the Magistrates ruled like this even flabbergasted our lawyer.

For us, leaving Barbara off the birth certificate had severe consequences since Amalia's Canadian Citizenship had to flow via Barbara's descent, as I am not a citizen of Canada, but a Permanent Resident. But perhaps more importantly, this was a huge emotional blow to Barbara. With everything we had battled as a couple to become parents, a judge in his ivory tower puts it into question whether or not Barbara should be considered a parent to Amalia.

In a twist of fate, this extremely conservative judge fell ill at the beginning of December. Apparently so ill that all cases were transferred to his Secretary (a vice-judge if you will). We took the opportunity to meet with this Secretary. He was much younger, clearly educated with perfect English, and an acting judge. I remember outlining all of these violations to him and that there was only one safe space for Amalia, back home in Canada.

We clearly made an impression on him because following this meeting, everything went smoothly and as expediently as possible.

We ended up with all of our paperwork, a birth certificate with Barbara and I as parents, and a Canadian passport for Amalia in February 2024. We decided to wait one more week before travelling back home so that Amalia could get her last set of vaccines before going on an airplane. At the beginning of March 2024, we flew back home with our little girl.

I have mostly very fond memories of our stay in Mexico City. Spending time with Bety and her family, as well as getting to know our egg donor better was wonderful. We made connections with other intended parents, some of whom we still keep in contact with to this day.

Almost two years have passed since we travelled home. As Santiago already predicted, most of the painful and stressful memories are gone. What remains is a lifetime of memories of all the beautiful aspects of this journey, and of course most importantly, our little Amalia.

From the Heart of Sam

OUR EGG DONOR

When I first heard about egg donation, it wasn't something I decided on immediately. I took the time I needed to reflect on it calmly. I researched, read, and sought information about the risks, how it could affect my body, and what it truly means to donate such an intimate part of oneself. I wanted to understand not only the medical process, but also the deeper meaning behind that decision.

After some time of reflection I began to see it from a different perspective. I realized it could be something very beautiful: the possibility of becoming part, in a very specific and conscious way, of another family's story. I thought about what it means to deeply desire a child and not be able to have one, and I put myself in the place of families who walk that path. I asked myself how I would feel if one day I were in that situation. I knew that if the roles were reversed, I would hope someone could help me fulfill such a meaningful dream. I also felt that this was a way of giving something good back to the world, of offering something genuine from myself. With that clarity and sense of peace, I made the decision to donate my eggs.

In 2022, I got in touch with Barbara and Koen. While we were getting to know each other, I was already familiar with the entire egg donation process and felt quite comfortable with it. We had a video call to meet one another, both them getting to know me and me getting to know them.

They asked me questions, and I asked questions as well. We talked about their lives, their story, and the situation they were going through. They shared with me the long journey they had already experienced, including processes such as adoption, driven by their deep desire to build a family and have a child. I remember thinking that what they went through was a long process that required a great deal of patience.

After that call, I was left with a very clear feeling. They are a couple of very genuine people. You can see that they have huge hearts full of love, very warm smiles, and a deeply familiar way of being. I connected with them from the very first moments in a natural and sincere way.

When we felt that both sides were happy, calm and comfortable with that connection and with the new bond that was forming, we decided to move forward. After a period of preparation, we were able to take the next step, which was to begin the medical treatment.

They were in Canada and I was in Mexico, so while they supported me from a distance, I attended the medical appointments. The doctor was always very kind, attentive, and friendly, which made everything feel much more manageable. Overall, the entire process was very pleasant and made me feel well cared for and supported.

The treatment consisted of daily hormonal injections to stimulate the ovaries in order to obtain the eggs. That was not the most enjoyable part. The treatment, in total, lasts approximately fifteen days, including the period of hormonal stimulation and the day of the extraction. The recommendations during that time are fairly standard: taking care of your diet, eating cleaner foods, avoiding irritating or very greasy meals to prevent discomfort and abdominal bloating, drinking plenty of water, and avoiding very intense exercise during the last days of treatment. Everything is quite manageable and a natural part of the process.

These injections eventually led to the day of the egg retrieval, which marks the final stage of the treatment: the moment when the eggs are extracted.

Throughout the entire medical process, Barbara and Koen were very attentive to me - checking in on how I was feeling, whether I needed anything, and how I was experiencing each stage. That constant support was very important to me. Especially on the day of the donation, I truly felt accompanied. It was a big surprise when Koen came to visit me at the clinic. Barbara couldn't be there that day due to work commitments, but even so, she was very present - attentive, involved, and accompanying the entire process, even from a distance. Koen brought me small gifts from Canada on behalf of both of them, a simple gesture but one full of affection. They are little keepsakes that I still have with me to this day. That gesture made me feel truly cared for, appreciated, and cherished. It's hard to put that emotion into words, but it was a warm, deeply human feeling - of living something meaningful alongside good people.

After the process was completed, we stayed in touch. They were always very attentive toward me, and from the very beginning there was a genuine interest and sincere communication on their part. We kept in contact while they began their own journey, which at that point was the pregnancy with Amalia. They were incredibly kind to me, always sending photos each month, sharing every stage with so much detail, care, affection, and love. They were deeply happy, and that happiness was contagious.

For me, it was very special to be included in that process. Living that moment alongside them, even from a distance, gave even more meaning to everything that had happened before.

When Amalia was finally born, everything took on an even deeper meaning. Meeting her was a very special experience for me. She is a sweet, joyful, intelligent little girl, full of life.

In some way, they made me feel like part of their family, from a place of deep respect and gratitude. Knowing that

I was able to contribute to something so important and so full of love left me with a sense of fulfillment that is hard to describe.

For me, it was an honor to have been a small part of such a beautiful process, to have been able to contribute something meaningful to a story filled with love, and to have been part of the realization of such a great dream. It is an experience I hold with affection, gratitude, and a deep sense of peace in my heart, and one I will carry with me always.

Today, I am very happy for them. Seeing the joy they share as a family, being the wonderful and incredible parents that they are, truly fills my soul. I know they hold me in their hearts, just as I hold them in mine. Today, that family is part of my life and my story, and they are people I am deeply proud to have in my life.

From the Heart of Santiago

OUR SURROGACY AGENCY OWNER IN MEXICO

I've been trying to find the right words to describe what Barbara and Koen mean to me, and honestly, it's not easy. In this work, you meet many families. You accompany them through one of the most vulnerable moments of their lives. Some families stay with you, and Barbara and Koen are one of those families.

When we first spoke, they had already been trying to have a baby for almost eight years. Eight years. Barbara had been diagnosed with diminished ovarian reserve and stage four endometriosis. IVF hadn't worked. Their doctor had told them that surrogacy with an egg donor was their only option. By the time they found us, they had already been through so much, and yet there was something in them that hadn't broken. A determination. A hope that refused to die.

What I remember most from those early conversations was how much they cared about doing things right. They didn't just want a baby. They wanted to know that the woman who would carry their child was being treated well, that she had chosen this freely, and that they could build a real relationship with her. That mattered to them. They asked about our ethical standards, about how we vetted surrogates, and about what kind of support we provided throughout the journey. That's when I knew these were special people.

Running a surrogacy agency means working with two groups of people whose lives will be forever intertwined: the intended parents who dream of having a child and the surrogates who offer their bodies and their hearts to make that dream possible. Our job is to protect both. To vet carefully. To match thoughtfully. To be there when things go wrong. Barbara and Koen understood this instinctively. They weren't looking for a transaction. They were looking for a relationship.

Then came Bety.

My best friend Salvador and I founded Gestacy in 2017. We'd been running a fertility consultancy in Spain for years, and we launched our Mexico program in 2021 with a very specific goal: to create an ethical, surrogate-centered alternative where women have their own lawyers, comprehensive medical care, life and medical insurance and 24/7 emergency support. Bety was our coordinator there. In April 2022, when Koen flew to Mexico City for the medical procedures, he met Bety at his hotel. Barbara joined via FaceTime. They clicked immediately. There was laughter, there was warmth, there was connection.

The next day, I received a message that changed everything: Bety wanted to be their surrogate.

This doesn't usually happen. Normally, matches are the result of weeks of careful work - reviewing profiles, video calls, deliberation. We vet surrogates rigorously: preliminary screenings, comprehensive applications, psychological evaluations, social work analysis, home visits and medical screenings at the fertility clinic. We need to know that she's doing this for the right reasons, that her family supports her, and that she understands what she's signing up for. But sometimes the universe intervenes. Sometimes two people meet, something clicks and you just know.

I still remember calling Barbara and Koen to tell them. The joy in their voices. After everything they had been through, here was this woman, who they had just met and already adored, offering to help them become parents. It felt like the universe was finally giving them a break.

The months that followed were full of legal paperwork, the kind of bureaucratic marathon that tests everyone's patience. But on January 11, 2023, the embryo transfer finally happened. Then came the waiting. Ten days that must have felt like ten years.

On January 24, Bety took the pregnancy test. Positive.

I wrote them an email that day. I think I just wrote "WOOOOOOW!" in capital letters. Because what else can you say? After eight years of heartbreak, they were finally pregnant.

The pregnancy went beautifully. In April 2023, Barbara and Koen traveled to Mexico City to visit Bety and her family. They spent time together, felt the baby kick and shared meals. This is what we encourage at Gestacy - the bond between intended parents and surrogate. Because surrogacy isn't a service you purchase; it's a relationship you build. When they came back, Barbara wrote to me that it had been "the most incredible trip of our lives." She said they missed Bety already. A journalist from Le Monde even interviewed them during that visit, wanting to tell their story. They said yes, because that's who they are. They wanted to help others understand that surrogacy can be something beautiful.

On September 15, 2023, at around 9:30 in the evening, Amalia was born. 3,050 grams. 49 centimeters. Perfect.

Barbara and Koen waited in Bety's room while the C-section was performed. Bety's husband Jesus took photos. And then, finally, they held their daughter.

"We are so happy and grateful and blessed," Barbara wrote to us that night.

I wish I could tell you that was the end of the story - that they flew home a few weeks later and lived happily ever after. But life doesn't always work that way.

The Mexican legal system had other plans.

What should have been a straightforward process to get both parents on Amalia's birth certificate turned into a nightmare. In early December the courts ruled that only Koen could be listed as a parent. Barbara, the woman who had dreamed of this child for eight years, who had endured countless medical procedures, who had poured her heart into this journey, was told she couldn't be on her own daughter's birth certificate.

Travel restrictions were imposed. They couldn't leave Mexico.

I remember reading Koen's emails during that time. The frustration. The disbelief. "It is honestly mind-boggling how little regard for the law these judges and magistrates have," he wrote. And he was right. It was mind-boggling. It was unfair. It was cruel.

This is the part of running an agency nobody talks about. The crises. The calls at midnight. The feeling of helplessness when you've done everything right and the system still fails your families. We arranged therapy sessions for them. I stayed in touch constantly, even though I felt helpless. There's only so much you can do when you're fighting a legal system that refuses to see reason.

Christmas 2023 came and went. Barbara and Koen spent it in Mexico City, far from their families in Calgary and Portugal. They had friends there, other intended parents going through similar journeys, and they made the best of it. But it wasn't home. Every day away from home, with their newborn daughter and an uncertain legal situation, took its toll.

But here's the thing about Barbara and Koen: they didn't give up. They didn't break.

Between Christmas and New Year's, they went to the courthouse. They asked to speak to the judge. Koen sat down with him and explained, calmly but firmly, what was happening to their family. He talked about their rights.

About Amalia's rights. About the need to go home.

Something shifted.

On January 8, 2024, the judge issued a new ruling. Both Barbara and Koen were listed as Amalia's legal parents. The relief was immense. Barbara cried. I think we all did a little.

Their lawyer said the ruling was "extraordinarily firm" in their favor. Every argument, every document, every plea had been heard. In 84 days, they had navigated what could have taken much longer. Koen joked that they had turned Court #4 into a "surrogacy-friendly court."

I met them in person for the first time in late January 2024, during a trip to Mexico City. After all those emails, all those calls, all those months of crisis, we finally shook hands. Hugged. It was emotional. Here were these two people who had been through hell and came out the other side with their dignity, their grace, and their humor intact.

On March 4, 2024, almost six months after Amalia's birth, they finally landed in Calgary. "We are finally back home." Barbara wrote. "What a journey it has been."

What a journey indeed.

But here's what I love most about Barbara and Koen. The story didn't end there.

They still talk to Bety every week. Every single week. They send photos of Amalia, now a toddler who, according to them, is "very spicy" and full of life. Bety sends updates about her own family. The bond they built during the pregnancy has only grown stronger. This is what surrogacy can be when it's done right. Not a transaction that ends at delivery, but a relationship that lasts a lifetime.

Barbara became an administrator of a support group for intended parents in Mexico. She spends hours helping strangers navigate the same fears and confusions she once faced. Koen writes detailed updates to help future families understand the legal process. They've done interviews, shared their story publicly and become advocates for surrogacy done right, including in November 2025 when *Fertility Matters Canada* featured their story.

In June 2025, when Amalia was 21 months old, they wrote to congratulate me on the birth of my own child. Just a simple, warm email asking how I was doing, telling me how much joy Amalia brought them every day. Koen wrote something that I will never forget: "The hurdles are long forgotten, and if it wasn't for you and your amazing team, we would not have this darling little girl that fills every day with so much joy. I can never thank you enough."

I read that email several times. Because the truth is, I should be thanking them.

In September 2025, Barbara and Koen told me they wanted to start their second journey. A sibling for Amalia. When I heard that, I felt a mix of honor and responsibility. After everything they went through, they trusted us again. They wanted to do it all over again.

"We would love to have a similar relationship with our new surrogate as we had with Bety," Barbara wrote. Because for them, surrogacy was never just about having a baby. It was about connection. About family, in the broadest, most beautiful sense of the word.

People ask me what it's like to run a surrogacy agency. The truth is, it's hard to explain. It's not the paperwork, the vetting protocols, or the legal battles - though all of that is essential. It's the moment when a family who has been through eight years of heartbreak finally holds their daughter. It's the calls between Calgary and Mexico City. It's the email you receive years later thanking you for making their life complete. Barbara and Koen taught me that.

Barbara and Koen, if you're reading this: thank you. Thank you for your patience when things were hard. Thank you for your kindness when you had every reason to be angry. Thank you for the way you treated Bety - the way you treat everyone - with such warmth and respect. Thank you for trusting us with your dream.

You taught me that resilience isn't just about surviving. It's about keeping your heart open even when life gives you every reason to close it. You taught me that the families we build through surrogacy are real families, with real bonds that last long after the legal papers are signed.

Amalia is so lucky to have you. And I am so lucky to know you.

The hurdles are long forgotten. What remains is love.

From the Heart of Katie

OUR EGG DONOR AGENCY OWNER IN CANADA

When I first met Barbara and Koen, what stood out right away was how thoughtful and intentional they were about becoming parents. Like many intended parents, they came to us holding both hope and uncertainty. Hope that this path could work and uncertainty about how it might unfold. From the beginning, our role was never just about coordinating logistics. It was about getting to know them, understanding what mattered to them, and supporting them as they worked toward building their family.

As they explored our donor database together, it didn't take long for them to identify an egg donor who felt like a genuine fit. One thing that has always mattered deeply to us at Her Helping Habit is prioritizing connection before any medical steps take place. Transparency matters in this process. These are real people and this is a lifelong story. Everyone deserves the opportunity to meet one another as humans, not just as profiles on a page.

One moment that stays with me most was introducing Barbara and Koen to their egg donor during a standard part of our process called the "meet-and-greet" call. These calls usually last about thirty minutes and take place before a match is finalized. They exist to give everyone space to see if things feel aligned emotionally, ethically and personally.

In many programs, intended parents don't meet their donor until after retrieval, if they meet at all. We've seen how that can unintentionally place donors on a pedestal or create expectations that don't always match reality. Sometimes profiles don't fully reflect the person behind them, and in some cases, profiles or photos may even be altered. Our approach is different. Intended parents deserve to know who is helping them build their family, and donors deserve the opportunity to meet the people they may be helping and feel empowered to say yes or no.

Barbara and Koen's call with their donor felt easy from the start. The conversation flowed naturally. There was warmth, openness and mutual respect. It was one of those moments where you can sense something meaningful taking shape, even before anything official happens. From there, we moved forward with the match sheet, counselling, legal steps and ultimately the medical process, knowing that care and understanding had been established early on. That foundation creates space for ongoing communication when needed, particularly around medical updates, and ensures donors can be informed when a birth takes place.

Mexico brought a different pace and a different set of considerations. Travelling for care, navigating another country's medical and legal systems, and building relationships across borders can feel overwhelming. Our role was to help create steadiness in that uncertainty during the egg donation process. We focused on clear communication and ensuring Barbara and Koen felt informed as decisions were made. We worked closely with their clinic, legal team, and our on-the-ground partners, while keeping Barbara, Koen and their donor fully informed at every step.

As the journey continued, Barbara and Koen met their egg donor in person. Those moments added an essential layer of grounding to the process and reinforced the trust that had already been established. Today, they remain in touch with her, and their daughter is growing up knowing the person who helped bring her into the world as a real individual, not an abstract figure. That continuity matters. It creates a foundation that can support a child not only at birth, but throughout her life.

At the time, our program in Mexico was still relatively new. I remain deeply grateful that Barbara and Koen trusted us with the egg donation process at a pivotal moment. Watching their story unfold has been a meaningful reminder of the impact this work can have long after the donation has concluded.

Their experience reinforces why we approach egg donation at Her Helping Habit the way we do, with transparency, respect, and a long-term view of the relationships created through donation. Supporting Barbara and Koen through their egg donation journey has been a true privilege. Their story is a reminder that when this part of the process is approached with care, intention, and humanity, it can create not only the foundation for a family but lasting connections built on trust.

Katie

Her Helping Habit

From the Heart of Abilio & Rebecca

A HOPEFUL FAMILY

I guess we will start at the beginning. My name is Abilio, I am forty-two years old and I'm married to the love of my life Rebecca, who is thirty-nine. We are an Australian couple currently undergoing surrogacy in Mexico City. We've been together since April 2011, and 2026 is our 15th year together. From the very beginning we were all in. Within a week or so we moved in together (kinda!). We both were living with our mums, or our mums were living with us. We began talking about marriage and having kids extremely early on, literally within our first month!

Despite never really being careful in terms of using contraception, we never got pregnant, but early on this did not really worry us.

As soon as we could, we moved in together and in September/October 2011 we got our own place. We got engaged in December 2012, although we had been planning for that a while before, and we married in July 2013. This was when we really started thinking about trying to have kids.

Our story, while it's been one of deep love for one another, together through thick and thin, has also been a tough one. From an early time, my wife has had several gynecological challenges, from being early diagnosed with abnormal pre-cancerous cervical cells and requiring LLETZ treatments, to suffering from polycystic ovarian syndrome (PCOS) and irregular periods.

During 2014 to 2015 however, it was very clear that something else started going wrong. My wife suffered from an extremely bad form of menorrhagia, one that was so bad that she bled every single day for an entire year.

Despite visiting five different public hospitals and gynecologists, undergoing various blood tests, taking all sorts of medication, scans and much more, no one could figure out what was going on. Her hormones were normal. Doctors ruled out fibroids, endometriosis and adenomyosis. We were told time and time again that what she was experiencing should not be happening.

This condition got so bad that it culminated in a visit to our General Practitioner in which we were asking to examine my wife's ongoing migraines and pains. The GP worryingly ordered an iron level blood test, which came back dangerously low. I remember our doctor saying that if she had come in two weeks later, she would probably be on her death bed or worse. We began iron infusions immediately.

Fed up with this, I lost hope in the public medical system that routinely ignored my wife's condition. They offered up such ridiculous treatment for a then twenty-eight year old, from Endometrial Ablations and Hysterectomies, both of which would leave her permanently infertile, in addition to also suggesting more D&C's. We sought a private gynecologist, who for the first time was able to shed light on what could actually be going on. His suggestions were to put my wife on an IUD called Mirena or alternatively attempt pregnancy via IVF. The latter would be too risky, however, since Rebecca was too unwell and her body was unlikely to survive a pregnancy at this stage.

Fortunately, the IUD worked its magic. Within a week my wife was feeling better than she had in years. Sadly, this meant a delay in our plan for having children by at least two years while we waited for her body to recover and bounce back to health. Our doctor did warn us that the condition could return should the IUD be removed, however this was unlikely to happen.

In 2018, we started planning to try again, remove the IUD, and work with our gynecologist to attempt pregnancy. Thankfully the condition did not return! My wife was put on various medications to help stimulate her ovaries and sadly after three cycles of medicated timed intercourse, this failed. Not for a lack of trying! One might think this sounds like a lot of fun, but deliberately trying to do this takes the joy out of it, and introduces a heck of a lot of stress and expectation.

At this point, our gynecologist suggested IVF, and that IUI would be unlikely to make much of a difference. With low sperm count of not amazing quality to begin with, IVF would provide a much higher chance of success.

We began this in March 2020, at the early beginnings of COVID-19, when lockdowns and restrictions descended upon us all. We started our treatment literally a week before our state government put restrictions on elective procedures and were fortunately allowed to continue. The hormone injections were brutal. Instant migraines, nausea, and dizziness took over and continued day after day, only getting worse as the cycle progressed. The doctor kept a close eye on my wife's treatment and the estradiol levels in her blood samples kept climbing. This was slightly concerning but the doctor was confident.

He suggested that we attempt a Fresh Embryo Transfer, which required a HCG trigger injection, as opposed to an egg collection for freezing, containing GnRH instead. We performed one final blood test the morning before the trigger shot. Sadly,this blood test was delayed due to backlogs in the lab caused by COVID-19 testing. The doctor was pretty sure that it would be ok to proceed with the HCG trigger, which we promptly carried out that evening.

When the doctor got the results the next day however, he noticed something was very wrong. The estradiol levels had jumped from 7000 pmol/L to well over 18,000 pmol/L, which was an extreme concern for Ovarian Hyperstimulation Syndrome (OHSS). At this point there was nothing anyone could do. The egg collection continued and we collected 31 eggs, and returned home. Sadly, things really went downhill from there. Rebecca began vomiting violently 3 days later, after not being able to go to the toilet, and was in excruciating pain. Terrified, we placed a 3am call to our doctor, who suggested we rush to hospital and meet him in the morning. COVID-19 protocols dictated I could not enter, and I left as I saw my wife walking into the emergency department of our hospital. Thirty minutes later, my wife calls me with really upsetting news; her kidneys were failing, her abdominal cavity had filled with fluid from her swollen ovaries and she was at risk of heart failure. As my wife was admitted into the hospital, I was able to join her in her room. To add insult to injury, as my wife spent her birthday in hospital, our first embryo count updates kept coming in, lower each day. Then a UTI set in, and we had to stay an extra day. A total of 4 days in hospital later, we were finally discharged, with the final kick to the teeth being that our large number of eggs dwindled down to two embryos. As expected, the fresh transfer was cancelled as it would have been too dangerous to continue.

As the months progressed, we attempted transferring some embryos to no avail. None would even take. Eventually however, during a very nasty flu, we performed a transfer and the embryo stuck. We were really hopeful! Sadly, this was short lived. As my wife recovered from the flu, she immediately miscarried, which made no sense whatsoever to us. It broke our hearts; we thought we had a baby on the way, but this ended at 7 weeks. At this point we'd committed to a total of four cycles, and we would give it one more shot, which sadly would fail to even implant.

As people often say, madness is trying the same thing over

and over again without a different result. So we changed doctors and clinics. Our new doctor decided to run a battery of tests to determine whether there were any reasons for the continuing infertility. Sadly, one of the results of these tests was a diagnosis of a genetic issue known as Major histocompatibility complex, class II, DQ alpha 1 (HLA-DQa1), also described as DQalpha by a lot of sufferers. Consults with a renowned reproductive immunologist would give us even worse news. The chances of a full match, of which we had been diagnosed with, meant that 100% of the time my wife's immune system would treat both my sperm and our embryos as cancerous cells and send Natural Killer Cells in the uterus to kill them. For the first time, we had a diagnosis and an explanation as to why, after more than 10 years, we had been unsuccessful in conceiving. This, however, meant that it was unlikely that we would be able to have a baby of our own genetics, unless someone else was able to carry it. The other options were donor sperm, or a fairly experimental immune protocol known as Lymphocyte Membrane Immunotherapy (LMIT), which also came with no guarantees, was also extremely expensive and not covered by insurance or the public healthcare system.

We decided instead to try donor sperm, and resigned to not being able to have our own fully biological child. We accepted this, because not having children at all was not a choice we were prepared to take. One would think though, that two vials of "man juice" would not have cost an arm and a leg, but $5000 USD later, express shipped to our clinic, they arrived. We began another IVF egg collection cycle and produced our best ever result - 6 embryos in a single cycle! I guess being young and virile really makes a difference! Sadly, out of the six embryos failed to take, with the very last attempt being 2 embryos in one attempt. That resulted in a miscarriage - our second one - right on Easter in 2024, while we were on holidays with friends.

It was at this point that we decided we had enough. My wife **<u>was not</u>** going to carry a baby to term. At this point we had done 7 IVF cycles and 9 embryo transfers and it was too much to bear the continual disappointment, pain and anguish. We turned to surrogacy after attending a surrogacy conference in our city and did two more IVF cycles and produced six embryos.

After long discussions we decided on Argentina. It fit us well. As an Australian and Portuguese citizen with eight years having lived in Portugal, I was fluent in Portuguese and fluent enough in Spanish to make it be some kind of crazy adventure and an opportunity to get better at it!

We believed the short timeframes for matching and the promise of a quick exit with both of us on the Birth Certificate were the ticket, in addition to being cheaper at the time than Mexico. We researched and found an agency that we liked. Our criteria was simple:

- We wanted transparency and fast communication - all other agencies we'd reached out to in Argentina were so slow - some didn't even get back to us!
- We wanted reasonably fast matching, we'd already waited twelve years at this point!
- We wanted to be able to talk to our surrogates and connect with them.
- We wanted to find a program where we could afford to have two babies at once, instead of doing multiple consecutive journeys.

We had also looked into Mexico, and we came close to selecting it, however the Amparo process seemed slow and scary and we aimed for Argentina instead. Sadly, as we got closer to shipping our embryos, the news started coming in about the Supreme Court in Argentina ruling that the surrogate must be recognised on the birth certificate. This would have wide ranging consequences for us as Australian citizens, as it would require us to wait until our children were

5 years old and go through a slow and expensive adoption process in Australia.

Thankfully, our agency had a plan, and pivoted to offering surrogacy journeys in Mexico. They previously had only offered other locations such as Colombia and Georgia, but neither of these appealed to us for a range of reasons. Columbia and Georgia both had legal uncertainty and there was uncertainty around production of birth certificates with both intended parents on it in Colombia at the time. Our Australian lawyer strongly advised us to pursue surrogacy in Mexico, as he had a litany of successful journeys from his clients there, and the process enjoyed strong constitutional protections for children born through surrogacy. We signed new contracts and began the process of preparing to ship our six precious embryos to Mexico.

Our agency worked quickly to ensure we would be matched quickly and even bent the rules a bit by allowing us to match while we were waiting to ship. We met our wonderful surrogates and our local coordinator in April via a Zoom call and decided to proceed.

As fate would have it though, the embryos never made it to their final destination, having suffered a catastrophic heat event. Another significant set back. Because having your heart broken a dozen times isn't enough, we had to endure yet more pain and suffering. Our surrogates were waiting, with insurance paid, we had a tough choice to make - quit, or fly to Mexico and spend 3 months making more embryos. This was not an easy decision, as there was so much at stake.

It wasn't just money; while that was a significant hurdle, and one that we would have to solve by borrowing money from the bank. It wasn't just the leave required, as my employer would not allow me to work overseas due to taxation reasons. My father-in-law had also been diagnosed with cancer in April, and we knew he would no longer be able to live by himself. We undertook a massive task to renovate his house so it could be rented out and simultaneously have a Granny Flat (as we call it in Australia, also known as an "in law suites" or Auxiliary Dwelling Units), and literally completed both within one week of our flight to Mexico.

At the time of writing this, we are in Mexico City. It has not been an easy time. For two out of the three months we've had significant hurdles, including spending most of that time in our apartment, as Rebecca suffered immensely under the hormone therapy treatments required for the egg collections. At one point even suffering severe abdominal impaction requiring hospitalisation as a result of a combination of factors. All in all our two cycles here were able to produce exactly seven embryos (one of which was aneuploid, and three of which are awaiting PGT-A testing results).

It would be remiss of me to miss the silver lining in our being here. During our three months here we were able to meet the wonderful professionals who would look after my wife, our journey coordinator, and our two generous and amazing surrogates. Better even, we got to meet their families and, in a strange sense, our new extended family. We've gotten to embrace them, share our story, get to know them and be inspired by their contribution to our lives.

So far we're early in this journey, and there's a lot of uncertainty and doubt, but not about the two courageous ladies who are carrying our hopes and dreams for a future we've been dreaming of for thirteen years, eleven IVF cycles, and seventeen lost embryos to time, and circumstances.

From the Heart of Ashley

A NEW MOTHER VIA SURROGACY

I was born with a very rare medical condition called MRKH. I didn't learn about it until I was around sixteen, and at the time I didn't grasp the true impact it would have on my future. I stayed positive - maybe even a little naïve - believing surrogacy would always be an easy, straightforward option when it came time to build my family. That hope was short-lived. Before we ever reached Mexico, we had already gone through the heartbreak of finding two surrogates, enduring five rounds of IVF, and experiencing six embryo transfers that resulted in three miscarriages. By the time we began exploring international options, we were carrying years of grief, disappointment, and fatigue.

After seven years of trying to build our family in Canada, we were emotionally exhausted. We'd been on the rematch list with our Canadian agency for more than two years with no progress, and each month felt heavier than the last. After one particularly difficult breakdown, I asked our agency point-blank if there were any other options. That was the first time they mentioned a relatively new Mexican program they believed might be worth exploring. For the first time in a long time, we felt a small spark of hope.

We quickly arranged a meeting with our lawyer, who introduced us to the agency in Mexico. From the very first conversation with the owner, we felt understood. He recognized everything we had been through and met us with compassion and confidence. Without overthinking it, we signed on almost immediately.

At first, we didn't want to send our embryos to Mexico. Instead, we found a doctor in Toronto who agreed to perform the transfer in Canada and allow our surrogate to travel up for the procedure. While we waited to be matched with a surrogate who had a passport, we worked closely with both clinics - Canadian and Mexican - to make sure everyone was aligned. In September 2023, we were finally matched. We clicked right away and started the legal process soon after. Getting the documents translated and finalized took much longer than expected - until January 2024 - but once everything was officially signed, we began preparing for our first transfer in March.

Ten days before our surrogate was supposed to fly to Canada, the Canadian government abruptly changed the visa requirements for Mexican travelers. Panic set in. I spent hours e-mailing members of parliament, calling immigration lawyers, and reaching out to anyone who might possibly help. A friend also began contacting political connections on our behalf. Eventually, a few members of parliament championed our issue and someone inside the immigration office stepped up to expedite things. It also helped that our surrogate worked for an embassy and could secure appointments faster than most - some wait times for fingerprinting were months long. Miraculously, her visa was approved on a Wednesday morning and she flew to Canada the very next day. For the first time, it really felt like things were finally coming together - that this time might truly be different.

We met our surrogate in person for the first time in Toronto. We spent four days together, sightseeing and getting to know each other, before the transfer on St. Patrick's Day. That first transfer didn't take. The disappointment was crushing. We had fought so hard just to get to that moment, but we tried again immediately. On May 15th, it worked.

Still, I didn't jump for joy. Even as the pregnancy progressed, I found myself waiting for the other shoe to drop. After nine years of heartbreak, it was hard to believe any of this could actually be happening. I avoided making a nursery. I didn't want a baby shower. I stayed guarded for as long as I could.

The first trimester was especially stressful. Because the transfer happened in Canada but our care continued in Mexico City, both doctors had to coordinate everything, including medications. Dosages and brand names differed between countries, and more than once we were scrambling at the last minute to find acceptable alternatives. Their clinical approaches also differed until the first trimester was complete, which added another layer of anxiety.

But we were deeply involved in the pregnancy. We were FaceTimed into every appointment, had monthly ultrasounds, and even did three 3D scans. Seeing our baby grow helped calm our fears, and after the first trimester, the next six months passed surprisingly quickly.

The one challenge we faced during that time was with the obstetrician. The first doctor insisted on a C-section from the very beginning, even though our surrogate had previously delivered naturally and wanted to try again. In Mexico, C-sections are extremely common, but this wasn't her preference, so we switched to another obstetrician who supported her wishes.

In the end, we induced labour on January 18th, and Presley was born at 12:01 a.m. on January 19th. After hours of labour, we did need to proceed with an emergency C-section because the baby was stuck. I was in the operating room the entire time and was able to do skin-to-skin contact immediately. Meanwhile, my husband had no idea she'd been born because he had no service in the waiting area. I held her for just two minutes before she was taken to the nursery for tests, but shortly after, the doctor quietly brought my husband in so he could meet her for the very first time.

After the birth, things initially went smoothly. Our lawyer filed for the birth certificate right away, and the court issued a temporary one almost immediately. Our biggest obstacle came from the civil registry office - they kept pushing our appointment farther out, not wanting to grant it until the end of March. Fortunately, our lawyer managed to get us squeezed in alongside another couple and we finally had her official birth certificate printed. We went straight to the embassy that same day to apply for her citizenship and temporary passport. Three days later, everything was approved and we were cleared to go home. In total, we spent about six and a half weeks in Mexico after the birth.

I will never forget the moment we boarded our first flight home. I just cried. After nine long years, we were finally bringing our little girl home. For the first time in almost a decade, I felt like I could finally breathe.

PART III
Your Journey

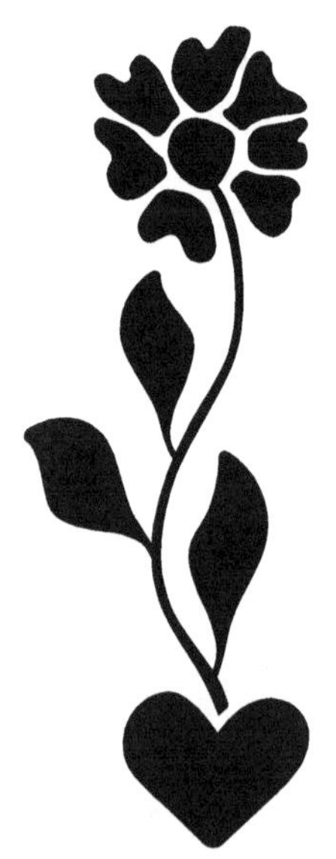

Your Surrogacy in Mexico Checklist

Legal

Surrogacy laws in Mexico vary by state. In Mexico City, surrogacy is legal, but there are specific legal laws that one must follow. At the time of this writing, the civil registry does not allow changes to the birth certificate due to the fact that the gestational surrogate is considered the mother and will be put on the birth certificate. This is when the legal team will step in and get the federal courts involved to sue the civil registry so that both intended parents can be on the birth certificate of the child. This is what is called an Amparo.

Procreational Will, which started in 2021, is when the Supreme Court of Mexico decided that anyone has a right to become a parent and is not adhered to by only genetics and who gives birth to the child. This is the will or intention to procreate of the intended parents.

The legal team files the Amparo in the federal court challenging the civil registry. There are 14 different courts available. The intended parents will be assigned one of these courts, they do not get to choose.

The judge will then look over the case, grant the Amparo and then order the civil registry to issue a new birth certificate with both intended parents on it.

This can be a lengthy process. Expect to be in Mexico City for two to three months on average, but this can fluctuate depending on which court the intended parents get.

Checklist of things to do:

- Hire a specialized surrogacy lawyer (bilingual recommended).
- Draft and notarize a surrogacy contract between intended parents and surrogate.
- Include clauses in that contract that specify parental rights at birth.
- Ensure contracts comply with Mexico City surrogacy laws.
- Prepare all identification documents: passports, birth certificates and marriage certificates (if applicable).
- File an Amparo with a legal team to secure parental rights.
- Confirm birth certificate issuance procedures before delivery.
- Have all documents translated and Apostilled (authentication of a legal document usually with a stamp) for use abroad.

Medical

Choose a clinic experienced in international surrogacy, with full transparency around procedures and success rates, and a strong ethical foundation in its practices.

Checklist of things to do:

- Select a reputable IVF clinic with surrogacy expertise.
- Confirm that surrogacy is legally allowed in that state.
- Sign medical contracts between all parties.
- Ensure complete medical and psychological screening for surrogate and intended parents.
- Oversee embryo creation and transfer schedule.
- Establish a prenatal care plan (regular checkups and ultrasounds).
- Confirm the delivery hospital and ensure it issues proper documentation.
- Arrange for newborn care (night nanny / pediatrician) and vaccinations.

Tips

- Request video consultations if you are abroad.
- Keep copies of all medical records for consular and embassy processes.
- Confirm the hospital's discharge policy for international surrogacy cases.

Agencies

Work only with transparent, licensed agencies that have verified success stories, clear financial terms, and a compassionate system that supports meaningful relationships with surrogates.

Checklist of things to do:

- Review and sign an agency contract (check inclusions carefully).
- Verify the agency's credentials and references.
- Understand the surrogate selection and screening process.
- Confirm details of egg/sperm donor programs and anonymity rules.
- Ensure clear payment schedules and milestone-based payments.
- Request regular progress reports during pregnancy.
- Verify insurance coverage for surrogate and baby.
- Arrange for post-birth support: paperwork, passport, and exit procedures.

Tips

- Consider hiring independent legal and medical experts, even if the agency offers them.
- Confirm surrogate support measures (medical, financial, psychological).

Practical

Planning your stay in Mexico ahead of time will save stress and ensure comfort during the birth and postnatal period.

Checklist of things to do:

- Book accommodation near the clinic/hospital (expect 2–3 months stay).
- Arrange transportation (airport transfers, daily rides with Uber).
- Get a local SIM card.
- Prepare baby essentials: diapers, formula, bottles, clothing, stroller, car seat. These can be bought in Mexico City or brought from your country.
- Bring or buy basic medical supplies: thermometer, hygiene products, baby meds.
- Find local grocery and pharmacy delivery options.
- Keep a list of emergency contacts: clinic, lawyer, embassy, translator.
- Prepare all travel documents for the baby: birth certificate, passport, consular appointment.
- Arrange translation services for the embassy (Spanish to English).

Tips

- Expect to stay 2-3 months after birth for paperwork and passport issuance especially when doing the Amparo.

- Have both cash and credit cards available for payments.
- Join local expat or surrogacy support groups for advice and resources.
- Use Uber for grocery delivery as well as for driving to appointments (legal and medical).

About the Author

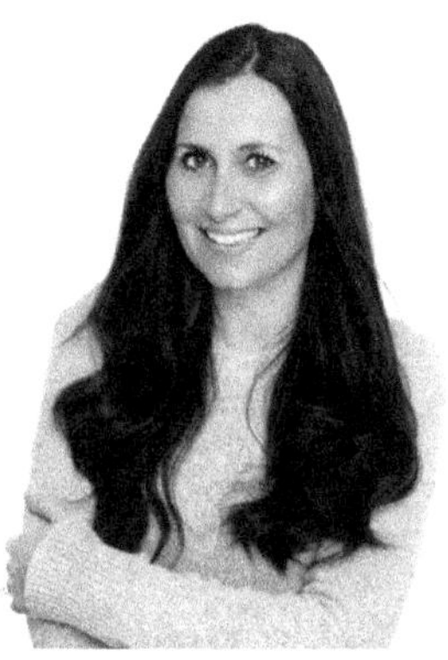

Barbara van der Maaten is a writer, advocate, and founder of Salsa & Surrogacy, a resource dedicated to helping intended parents navigate the complexities of international surrogacy and egg donation in Mexico. After a seven-year struggle with infertility, Barbara became a first-time mother through surrogacy and donor eggs, an experience that transformed her life and inspired her to support others on similar paths. Through Salsa & Surrogacy, she offers guidance, support, and firsthand insights for families considering or embarking on a surrogacy journey abroad, answering both the big questions and the small ones with compassion and clarity.

www.ingramcontent.com/pod-product-compliance
Lightning Source LLC
LaVergne TN
LVHW010837120826
845149LV00017B/1479

* 9 7 9 8 9 9 8 8 8 5 8 4 6 *